MAKING SENSE OF RESEARCH
IN NURSING, HEALTH & SOCIAL CARE

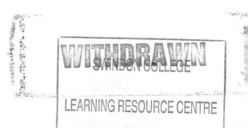

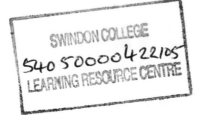

SAGE was founded in 1965 by Sara Miller McCune to support the dissemination of usable knowledge by publishing innovative and high-quality research and teaching content. Today, we publish more than 750 journals, including those of more than 300 learned societies, more than 800 new books per year, and a growing range of library products including archives, data, case studies, reports, conference highlights, and video. SAGE remains majority-owned by our founder, and after Sara's lifetime will become owned by a charitable trust that secures our continued independence.

Los Angeles | London | Washington DC | New Delhi | Singapore

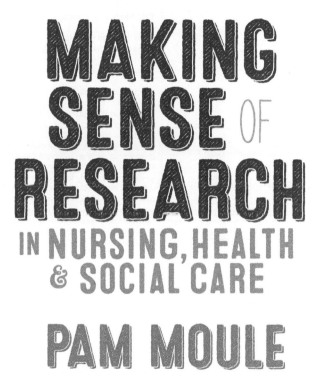

5TH EDITION

MAKING SENSE OF RESEARCH

IN NURSING, HEALTH & SOCIAL CARE

PAM MOULE

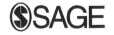

Los Angeles | London | New Delhi
Singapore | Washington DC

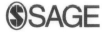

Los Angeles | London | New Delhi
Singapore | Washington DC

SAGE Publications Ltd
1 Oliver's Yard
55 City Road
London EC1Y 1SP

SAGE Publications Inc.
2455 Teller Road
Thousand Oaks, California 91320

SAGE Publications India Pvt Ltd
B 1/I 1 Mohan Cooperative Industrial
Area
Mathura Road
New Delhi 110 044

SAGE Publications Asia-Pacific Pte Ltd
3 Church Street
#10-04 Samsung Hub
Singapore 049483

Editor: Becky Taylor
Associate editor: Emma Milman
Production editor: Katie Forsythe
Copyeditor: David Hemsley
Proofreader: Sarah Cooke
Marketing manager: Tamara Navaratnam
Cover design: Wendy Scott and Perry Williams
Typeset by: C&M Digitals (P) Ltd, Chennai, India
Printed and bound by CPI Group (UK) Ltd,
Croydon, CR0 4YY

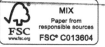

MIX
Paper from
responsible sources
FSC
www.fsc.org   FSC® C013604

First edition published by Continuum in 1996

Second edition published by Continuum in 2002.
Reprinted by SAGE Publications in 2003

Third edition published 2006. Reprinted 2007

Fourth edition published 2011. Reprinted 2011

This edition first published 2015

Library of Congress Control Number: 2014948467

British Library Cataloguing in Publication data

A catalogue record for this book is available from
the British Library

ISBN 978-1-4739-0752-2
ISBN 978-1-4739-0753-9 (pbk)

At SAGE we take sustainability seriously. Most of our products are printed in the UK using FSC
papers and boards. When we print overseas we ensure sustainable papers are used as measured
by the Egmont grading system. We undertake an annual audit to monitor our sustainability.

CONTENTS

LIST OF TABLES

LIST OF FIGURES

ABOUT THE AUTHOR

Pam Moule is Professor of Health Services Research and Director of the Centre for Health and Clinical Research at the University of the West of England, Bristol. Pam is engaged in a number of research and evaluation projects across a range of health care environments, supported by a variety of funders.

Pam delivers research methods education, supervises undergraduate and masters level dissertations, and supports Doctoral students in the fields of leadership, learning and workforce. Pam has a number of publications in a range of nursing and medical journals and has published four textbooks. Pam is on the editorial board of *Nurse Education Today* and reviews papers for a number of nursing and health care journals.

PREFACE

This book is intended for qualified nurses, health and social care practitioners and students who have limited understanding or experience of research. It is an introductory text designed to be of practical use for the practitioner of today. The aim is to 'demystify' and explain research by introducing the essential elements relevant to nursing and health and social care professionals.

The idea and motivation for the book came from experiences of teaching research awareness to pre-registration students and qualified practitioners on various courses. The book is clearly aimed at giving health and social care practitioners and students an introduction to research with the expectation that those practitioners wanting to 'do' research, will gain research training and read more in-depth and definitive texts to help them.

This fifth edition includes as its readership within the health and therapy professions, nurses, midwives, physiotherapists, radiographers, occupational therapists, speech and language therapists and paramedics. Within social care, the text is mainly directed at social workers and social work students as the primary group concerned with professional practice and decision-making across a range of social care needs. Statutory, voluntary and non-profit health and social services across primary, community, hospital and residential care have been considered, as well as social enterprise and private health care providers.

Policy documents have been closely examined and the book supports the view that the health and social care practitioners need to be 'research literate' and 'research aware'. Concepts such as 'evidence-based practice' and some of the issues and challenges faced by practitioners are introduced. A foundation for developing research knowledge and a basis for the critical appraisal of research is presented. Through this knowledge, the book is intended to help practitioners make sense of it all and enable them to become 'critical consumers of research'. This in turn will empower them to provide the highest standards of care for the public.

The layout of the book is straightforward and each chapter can be read on its own without the need to continually refer to other chapters. Following the first chapter that provides an overview of evidence-based practice and research in practice, and Chapter 2 that explores the nature of knowledge, Chapter 3 explores the research process, with further detail given in Chapters 5–10. Chapter 4 considers the important area of ethics in research and Chapter 11 is a key chapter that considers critical appraisal of research. The final chapter looks at the complex issues related to the dissemination and implementation of research into practice.

Three appendices are provided as useful resources for practitioners, and a glossary that defines appropriate research concepts. Each chapter has learning outcomes, key concepts, a list of suggested further reading and key websites. References for publications referred to in each chapter, some expanded and discussed, will be found in the reference list at the end of the book.

It is intended that this book will make research interesting for practitioners, and that it will stimulate further exploration of the subject. More importantly, it is designed to help practitioners understand and 'make sense of research' so that they can consider it in their daily practice. Members of the public using health care services can benefit from practitioners who are able to use research appropriately, and provide the highest standards of care possible. This is the ultimate aim of the book.

ACKNOWLEDGEMENTS

In this fifth edition of *Making Sense of Research* I would like to acknowledge the major contributions made to previous editions by the late Gill Hek, who was an inspiring nurse researcher and is greatly missed. I am also indebted to Maggie Judd who made significant contributions to the earlier editions of the book.

I am also grateful to a range of health and social care students and practitioners who continue to influence the style and content of this book. Their need to understand research as a practical activity has informed the ongoing development of the text, which presents practical examples of real relevance to the health and social care professionals of today.

SAGE Publications and I would like to thank the reviewers who commented on the fourth edition of this text: Nerys Bolton, Senior Lecturer in Adult Nursing and Critical Care at Canterbury Christ Church University; Dr June Keeling, Senior Lecturer at the University of Chester; Andrea Lacey, Lecturer in the School of Health and Social Care at Bournemouth University and Bernard Pennington, Senior Lecturer at Edge Hill University

Finally, thanks go to health and social care colleagues, and my family, who have supported me in writing this fifth edition.

ABOUT THE COMPANION WEBSITE

Visit http://study.sagepub.com/moule for access to a wealth of resources to support your studies and teaching if you are a lecturer.

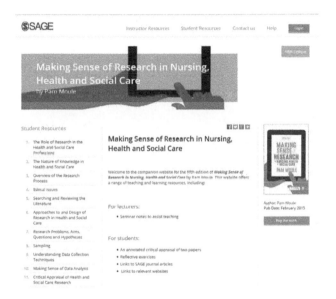

The companion website includes:

For students

- Reflective excercise related to each chapter of the book to help your understanding. These are linked to free SAGE journal articles, which can be used as examples of research and will expand your knowledge.
- A template critical appraisal framework to use in your own studies.
- A completed critical appraisal of a paper to use as an example.
- Weblinks to further resources.

For lecturers

- A lesson plan on critical appraisal of research.
- All the practice examples from the book for you to download and use in your teaching.

1 THE ROLE OF RESEARCH IN THE HEALTH AND SOCIAL CARE PROFESSIONS

LEARNING OUTCOMES

On completion of this chapter the reader should be able to:

- understand the development of research in the health and social care professions
- appreciate the need to become 'research literate'
- identify the major factors that contribute to debates about the nature of research and evidence
- understand the emergence and development of evidence-based practice
- consider different ways of defining research
- appreciate the economic costs associated with research activity.

KEY CONCEPTS

- research literacy
- evidence-based practice
- research in context

- research capacity and capability
- definitions of research
- hierarchies of evidence

INTRODUCTION

The terms 'research literate' or 'research aware' have been used by many to describe the way that the professional health and social care practitioner should be in the twenty-first century. These are the terms that are favoured here as the intention in this introductory book is not to provide a text that equips health and social care professionals to undertake research, but rather to assist all practitioners to become 'research literate' or 'research aware' through a greater understanding of research within their respective professional groups. However, this does not mean that health and social care practitioners should not be undertaking research. To the contrary, health and social care professions all need more research-ers in their field of practice and it is important to build the research capability (skills) of practitioner researchers as well as research capacity (volume). However, particular skills and knowledge are required to become a researcher in a particular field of practice, for example, social work, midwifery, physiotherapy, nursing, just as in any other specialist area, such as mental health, safeguarding chil-dren or cancer care, and that is beyond the remit of this book.

The majority of health and social care practitioners do not have, nor necessarily need, the skills required to undertake a research project themselves. What we all need, however, are the skills and knowledge to appreciate, understand and use research and evi-dence in order to provide the highest quality and most effective care possible for our patients, clients, service users and carers. It should be a natural activity for health and social care practitioners to keep up to date and use research findings and evidence in their work, and being 'research literate' is one of the basic skills required of all these professional groups.

RESEARCH LITERACY

The term 'research literate' means: having the capability for criti-cal thought, possessing analytical skills, having the skills to gain access to relevant research and evidence, having a critical under-standing of research processes, and being able to read and **criti-cally appraise** research and other types of evidence. Through possessing these skills and being research literate, health and social care practitioners will be able to assess the appropriateness of using specific evidence in their daily practice, and identify research problems and priorities. This is not an easy task and it is generally accepted that more health and social care practitioners need to become 'research aware' and 'research literate'.

Health and social care practitioners also need to have an aware-ness of any potential ethical issues that may arise in relation to their patients, clients, service users and carers if research is under-taken. This includes having an understanding of the implications of collecting data for other researchers, and the statutory duties and responsibilities associated with their professional groups that may not sit comfortably with research.

The groups that fall within the scope of health care and therapy professions that have been included in this book are nurses, midwives, physiotherapists, podiatrists, occupational therapists, speech and language therapists, radiographers, and paramedics. Within social care, social workers are considered as the primary group concerned with skilled delivery of a professional practice. These health and social care professional groups span: hospital, residential, community and primary care; statutory, voluntary, independent and non-profit health and social services; and preventive, therapeutic and supportive services.

Prior to the introduction of diploma and graduate level prequalifying education for many of these professional groups in health and social care, research awareness and understanding were limited in the curriculum. This means that there are many qualified practitioners who have not had the opportunity to explore and become aware of research and **evidence-based practice**. These practitioners now recognise the need to become 'research literate' and are seeking out opportunities to develop their understanding and awareness of research in the health and social services. There are many courses, study days, online and web-based resources, virtual groups and networks, books and journal articles which are more accessible to most practitioners, and being able to attend a conference or specialised study day is also a good opportunity to become aware of research in one's own area of practice.

The care provided by all health and social care practitioners must be based on current knowledge and evidence that promotes the delivery of the highest standards of care possible. All the professional groups in health and social care are working hard to develop their own professional knowledge base with strong foundations built on research and evidence. Each professional group has research leaders who are striving to develop research knowledge and evidence for both their professional colleagues and the users of their services, such as clients and patients. Excellence in practice is dependent on the research and evidence base of each professional group and we all have a responsibility in some way to contribute to our own profession's knowledge through research.

RESEARCHERS IN HEALTH AND SOCIAL CARE

As previously mentioned, there are many people who undertake research that could come under the broad category of health and social care research. There are those in disciplines such as psychology, sociology, social and welfare policy, and other social sciences who have a clear relationship with health and social care and who research from the perspective of their own discipline using techniques that might be specifically related to that discipline. There are also researchers, such as historians, economists, statisticians, epidemiologists, geographers and anthropologists, who will again bring their own discipline to a particular research project. Practitioners also undertake research from their own professional perspective, such as physiotherapy, social work or nursing, in order to make a direct improvement to their practice and this may involve more active research approaches than in other areas of research. Practitioners who are working in therapy or nurse consultant roles, or those who are advanced practitioners, are also likely to be undertaking research directly related to their area of expertise.

There is a growing body of service user and carer-led research that brings a different perspective to the research endeavour and an increasing attention to engaging service users in research activity. The engagement and involvement of the public in research is supported by the work of Involve (www.invo.org.uk). Involve is a national advisory group funded by the National Institute for Health Research (NIHR). Its role is to promote public involvement in NHS, public health and social care research. It supports the involvement of the public in research as it believes engagement makes the research more relevant, reliable and more likely to be used. The public are more often involved as co-applicants on research bids and can have various roles within the research. These may range from offering advice from the user perspective through to being a member of the research team with responsibility for various stages of the research, including data collection and analysis. This type of research and the researchers on the team will be seeking to directly improve care within a particular client or patient group.

There is a growing emphasis in health services research that requires the involvement of multidisciplinary teams to address **research questions**. These teams include health professionals, social scientists, statisticians and health economists. There may be physiotherapists, nurses, podiatrists or speech and language therapists directly employed in specialities such as carer support, breast care, respiratory medicine, paediatrics or diabetes care, who undertake small studies in their own area of work; or there may be health and social care practitioners employed directly on a specific project, for example a clinical trial examining the effectiveness of a counselling service, or looking at what works in family support. A quick look at journals related to the health and social services will give some idea of the types of research that are conducted and reported by health and social care professionals.

Some health and social care practitioners may undertake research as part of a pre- or post-qualifying degree course, or during a period of learning, and many more now study at postgraduate level including master's and doctoral studies. In 2005, for example, it was noted that 900 nurses were registered on doctoral programmes (Higher Education Statistics Agency, 2005). Health and social care students studying at diploma and degree level are often not encouraged to undertake research, although they might perform activities, such as designing a **questionnaire** or interviewing colleagues, as exercises to help them understand research methods. More commonly they will develop skills to enable them to critically appraise research in order to inform their practice and service improvement. Students may also undertake project work or write essays using research findings and evidence. All these activities are important and necessary in helping health and social care practitioners to become research literate.

Recently a commission on nursing has promoted the need for innovation in nursing and midwifery, promoting the need for capacity building, the development of research skills and strengthening the integration between nursing practice, education and research (Commission on Nursing and Midwifery, 2010). The changes to the provision of undergraduate nursing degrees only and the development of Clinical Academic Training Programme for Nurses, Midwives and Allied Health Professions (www.nihrtcc.nhs.uk) should further aid capacity building.

Health and social care practitioners are also being engaged in developing evidence-based quality care as part of the service improvement agenda for the NHS (Darzi, 2008; NHS Improvement, 2008). The service improvement approach takes a patient focus and reviews care delivery systems and processes in order to improve service delivery. Proposed care delivery changes are tested through a Plan, Do, Study, Act (PDSA) cycle. The cycle starts with a planned change, the change is implemented, and the outcomes are studied and used to inform further change **implementation**.

THE DEVELOPMENT OF EVIDENCE-BASED PRACTICE

Evidence-based practice has rapidly emerged since the early 1990s and has had a significant impact on health and social service provision. As the starting point for this movement, evidence-based medicine was seen as using its current evidence base to inform decisions about individual patient care, and the best evidence was not restricted to **Randomised controlled trials** (RCTs) (Sackett et al., 2006). There has been a swift adoption of key concepts in other professional groups, which are now using the terms evidence-based nursing, evidence-based occupational health, evidence-based public health and evidence-based mental health. In other areas, such as social work, the notion of evidence-based practice has been refashioned to reflect the need for social care professionals to research their practice and develop knowledge in ways that are appropriate for professional practice.

The growth of evidence-based practice is not without its critics across all areas of health and social care, and there is limited consensus on its merits. Some point out that there is no 'evidence' that evidence-based practice actually works and that it constrains professional decision-making and autonomy. It is criticised for being 'too simple'; and some argue that it is a covert method of rationing resources, that it exalts certain types of research evidence over other forms of knowledge and evidence and that research trials are not usually transferable (Janicek, 2006). Health and social care practitioners need to be aware of the debates surrounding evidence-based practice both within their own professional group and more generally in the health and social services.

The successful and rapid emergence of evidence-based practice has been attributed to the obvious, simple, sensible and rational idea that the most up-to-date, valid and reliable research should inform and be the foundation for practice (Melynk and Fineout-Overholt, 2005). The context in which it has developed may go some way to explain why the movement has been flourishing in many areas of health and social care practice. In recent years there has been a cultural shift within the health and social services from trusted professional judgement-based practice to evidence-based practice. Glicken (2005) and others suggest that there are a number of contributing factors in the development of evidence-based practice, including:

- growth in an increasingly well-educated and well-informed public
- increasing awareness of the limitations of science
- growth in consumer and self-help groups
- intensive media scrutiny
- an explosion in the availability of different types of information and data
- developments in information technology
- increasing emphasis on productivity and competitiveness
- emphasis on 'value for money' and audit
- increase in scrutiny, accountability and regulation of professional groups
- major adverse events within the health and social services
- lawsuits and compensation claims.

This cultural shift has resulted in an explosion of evidence-based initiatives and new terminology within the health and social services since the mid-1990s including:

- centres such as Evidence-based Mental Health, Evidence-based Nursing Practice, Research in Practice for Adults, Social Care Institute for Excellence (SCIE)
- specialist 'evidence-based' journals
- websites and web-based discussion lists
- electronic bibliographic resources for evidence-based practice.

This has had an effect on how research and evidence are considered and used by current practitioners within health and social care and how evidence and practice drive (and are driven by) practice and policy more than ever before.

Within the health and social services, political ideology plays a role in shaping both policy and practice. This can influence how health and social problems are perceived, problems solved, and services delivered by different professional groups. The professional groups work across organisations more than in the past, and joint working within and between many areas of health and social services means that communication and collaboration need to be effective if patients, clients and service users are to receive the highest quality of care. The development of public health services and the growing shift towards community and primary care have also had a role in the development of evidence-based initiatives. It is reasonable to say that the evidence-based practice movement has had an effect all through the health and social services including practice, policy, management and education, and that it includes all health and social care professionals who make decisions.

WHAT IS EVIDENCE-BASED PRACTICE?

There are three key components to evidence-based practice:

1. Best available current evidence.
2. Preferences of individual clients and patients.
3. Expertise and experience of the professional.

All three elements need to be used together, although the importance of each may vary in different situations. The overriding principle is that of giving the most effective care to maximise the quality of life for an individual. It should also be noted that evidence-based practice promotes quality and cost-effective outcomes of health care (Schmidt and Brown, 2011).

Evidence-based practice is seen as comprising five explicit steps:

1. Identify a problem from practice and turn it into a specific question. This might be about the most effective intervention for a particular client, or an assessment of causation, or about the most appropriate test, or about the best method for delivering a service.
2. Find the best available evidence that relates to the specific question, usually by making a thorough search of the literature.
3. Appraise the evidence for its **validity** (closeness to the truth), usefulness (practical application) and methodological rigour.
4. Identify current best evidence and, together with the patient or client's preferences, apply it to the situation.
5. Evaluate the effect on the patient or client, and the practitioner's own performance.

Current pre-qualifying education will help students address all these stages. Specifically practitioners need to learn how to search effectively for appropriate evidence and research through a range of literature sources (see Chapter 5), and how to critically appraise research (see all chapters, but particularly Chapter 11 and Appendix 3).

WHAT COUNTS AS EVIDENCE?

There are many debates and arguments across all the health and social care professions about what constitutes evidence. For the purposes of this book, research (defined later) is viewed as one form of evidence amongst many other types. Health and social care professionals should be aware of the debates surrounding types of evidence including research, and in particular hierarchies of evidence. The idea of a 'hierarchy of evidence' has evolved as a response to the notion that some research designs, particularly those using quantitative methods, are better able than others to provide robust evidence of effectiveness, that is, what works. The most common type of hierarchy (see Table 1.1) places randomised controlled trials (RCTs) at the top of the hierarchy.

Other chapters in this book guide the reader through some of these research designs, and the 'further reading' at the end of this chapter points to some useful texts that introduce the debates surrounding types and hierarchies of evidence. Of particular importance are the debates surrounding the role of experimentation and randomised controlled trials in social care, which, in health, have been seen as the 'gold standard' of research design for looking at effectiveness of interventions (see, for example, Davies et al., 2000; Trinder and Reynolds, 2000). As is evident later, hierarchies of evidence of effectiveness are only helpful for considering evidence about whether something works, such as a treatment, therapy or educational programme. Evidence about how clients feel about something, or whether patients are satisfied, or the perspective of different types of practitioners, is best captured by different types of research and evidence that do not particularly feature in any type of hierarchy. Furthermore, as will be seen in Chapter 2, evidence can be based on different types of knowledge, of which some types are more robust and systematic than others.

Table 1.1   *A basic hierarchy of strength of evidence about effectiveness (what works)*

1   Evidence from a systematic review of multiple well-designed randomised controlled trials.
2   Evidence from one or more well-designed randomised trials.
3   Evidence from trials without randomisation or from single before-and-after studies, cohort, time series or matched case-controlled studies or observational studies.
4   Evidence from well-designed descriptive studies or qualitative research.
5   Opinions from expert committees or formal consensus methods such as the National Institute for Health and Care Excellence (www.nice.org.uk).
6   Expert opinion.

See Evidence Based Nursing Practice at www.ebnp.co.uk for further examples.

The importance of nursing research for evidence-based practice has been reiterated in the recent Francis Inquiry (2013). The inquiry reviewed the care delivered at one NHS hospital and reinforced the need for National Institute for Health and Care Excellence (formerly known as the National Institute for Clinical Excellence)(NICE) evidence to inform evidence-based procedures and practices. In addition, it made a number of recommendations to improve care delivery including better complaints procedures and the need for improvements in supporting patient safety. Research evidence is used in the development of NICE guidance (www.nice.org.uk) which relates to a number of areas of clinical practice. The guidance is used to guide the delivery of up-to-date care and best practice and has the potential to reduce unnecessary costs and aid decision-making.

DEFINITIONS OF RESEARCH

There are many ways of defining research, ranging from very broad to narrow interpretations that often reflect the perspective of those undertaking the research. For example, the Department of Health (DH) defines research as 'the attempt to derive generalisable new knowledge by addressing clearly defined questions with systematic and rigorous methods' (DH, 2005: 3). This definition reflects a concern to undertake systematic and rigorous research to generate findings that can be used beyond the immediate area of research; in other words, that can be generalised. The focus on a systematic approach to research is one of the common elements seen in a range of research definitions. Most definitions of research include at least one of the following dimensions:

- a systematic approach to the enquiry
- a focus on developing existing or creating new knowledge
- activities that are planned and logical
- a search for an answer to a question.

Additionally, definitions may refer to the multidisciplinary nature of research and the need to use different research approaches. The scope of research can also be included in the definition, making reference to the generation of knowledge for practice, education and policy.

The definition of research provided in the first edition of this book remains relevant today:

> a systematic approach to gathering information for the purposes of answering questions and solving problems in the pursuit of creating new knowledge about health and social care.

This definition is broad in order to encompass all aspects of health and social care and it recognises the systematic nature of collecting data. In addition, the active, practical and applied nature of health and social care practice is considered. In order to distinguish research from audit, service improvement and development work, which are closely related, research is defined as creating new knowledge.

No single definition will be satisfactory, however, and in order to be able to understand research at an introductory level, it was felt that a working definition might be helpful. Chapter 2 considers how the research and evidence used in decision-making by practitioners is informed by different types of knowledge available to the practitioners.

RESEARCH FUNDING IN HEALTH AND SOCIAL CARE

The funding of health and social care research is driven by economic, political and organisational factors (Moule and Goodman, 2014). Research activity is expensive and is influenced by funding priorities. In the United Kingdom the NHS Research and Development strategy aims to maximise the benefits of scientific research for health. As part of the strategy, research and development offices were set up across the UK. They are funded by, and responsible to, the government for identifying NHS research needs and commissioning research to meet these needs. The National Institute for Health Research (NIHR) commissions and funds NHS, social care and public health research in order to develop research evidence to support professionals, policy makers and patients. Evidence is disseminated through NHS Evidence (www.evidence.nhs.uk) and through NICE. The translation of research into practice is also the role of the Academic Health Science Networks (www.england.nhs.uk). Their goal is to improve patient and population health outcomes by networking across health care providers, industry and academia to support collaborative working that will enable rapid evaluation and adoption of research and innovation.

Other major funders include charities, such as the Wellcome Trust (www.wellcome.ac.uk) who fund biomedical and human research, and funding councils such as the Economic and Social Research Council (www.esrc.ac.uk), the UK's leading agency for research funding in economic and social sciences. Health care staff are often part of teams who bid for funds from a wide range of charities and other funders; however, the application processes are highly competitive and success rates can be low.

KEY POINTS

- All health and social care practitioners need to become 'research literate'.
- 'Research literacy' includes the skills and knowledge to appreciate, understand and use research.
- Not all health and social care practitioners should be conducting research as part of their daily work or professional development.

(Continued)

(Continued)

- Health and social care practitioners need to consider the tensions and conflict associated with the concept of evidence-based practice.
- There are many definitions of research, with most incorporating a view about the search for knowledge through a systematic and rigorous process.
- Health and social care practitioners need to become critical consumers of research to enable them to provide excellence in care.
- Health and social care practitioners need to be aware that research takes place within a broad political and financial context.

FURTHER READING

Brett, J., Staniszewska, S., Mockford, C., Seers, K., Herron-Marx, S. and Bayliss, H. (2010). *The PIRCOM study: A systematic review of the conceptualisation, measurement, impact and outcomes of patient and public involvement in health and social care research.* London: UKCRC.

Cullum, N., Ciliska, D., Haynes, B. and Marks, S. (eds) (2007). *Evidence based nursing: An introduction.* Oxford: John Wiley and Sons.

Schmidt, N. and Brown, J. (2011). *Evidence based practice for nurses* (2nd edn). Sudbury, MA: Jones and Bartlett.

WEBSITES

Centre for Evidence Based Medicine: www.cebm.net
Centre for Reviews and Dissemination: www.york.ac.uk/inst/crd/
Department of Health: www.dh.gov.uk
Economic and Social Research Council: www.esrc.ac.uk
Evidence Based Nursing Practice: www.ebnp.ac.uk
Involve: www.invo.org.uk
NHS Improving Quality: www.nhsiq.nhs.net
UK Clinical Research Collaboration: www.ukcrc.org
Wellcome Trust: www.wellcome.ac.uk

2 THE NATURE OF KNOWLEDGE IN HEALTH AND SOCIAL CARE

LEARNING OUTCOMES

On completion of this chapter the reader should be able to:

- identify the sources of knowledge available to the health and social care professions
- appreciate the importance of research and evidence-based knowledge for health and social care practice.

KEY CONCEPTS

- sources of knowledge
- authority
- personal knowledge
- common sense
- tradition
- scientific knowledge

- rituals
- reflective practice
- trial and error
- tacit knowledge
- intuition

INTRODUCTION

Within this text the development of knowledge and practice, and the significance of research and evidence-based information to the nature of knowledge, are considered. It is the intention of this chapter to discuss how health and social care knowledge has developed, and to highlight the need for the health and social care professions to develop information as part of professional growth.

In an attempt to understand the nature of health and social care knowledge, the complexity of health and social care information is discussed and the multidimensional aspects of the profession's **theory** base are considered. The chapter will consider the importance of **evidence-based practice**, as identified in Chapter 1, specifically exploring the development of knowledge through **tradition**, ritualistic practice, **intuition, tacit knowledge, common sense**, authority, **trial and error**, and from a scientific base. Such discussions will reveal the many dimensions of health and social care theory, and, whilst not denigrating the development of any particular source of knowledge, will demonstrate the need for health and social care practitioners to question the underpinning knowledge base and accept those sources that provide a credible evidence base for practice. Thus, the practitioner might access a variety of forms of best evidence on which to base practice.

TRADITIONS AND RITUALS

'We do it this way because we believe this is the best way.' 'We do it the way the team leader likes it.' 'Dr X likes his patients to be treated in this particular way.' These statements reflect the use of tradition in the health and social care professions, the development of practice based on beliefs or myths which are accepted by the profession as a base for practice. Traditions can become customs, applied without critical thought, in a ritualistic way.

Traditions and **rituals** can impinge on all aspects of the patient's day and demonstrate the use of outdated practice by many nursing staff. Examples might include the ritual practice of recording observations of temperature, respiration, pulse and blood pressure without a clear rationale.

It should be noted, however, that certain routine practices, which might be seen as ritualistic, are not necessarily undesirable. The performance of the handing over of client information from one staff member to another might be part of the care routine, but can also act as a vehicle for social exchange and enhances social cohesion and team working.

Whilst some ritualistic practices might be beneficial, it is vital that outdated and unsafe practices are identified to allow health and social care practitioners to feel confident in the delivery of safe practice. As new evidence emerges there is a need to challenge and change traditional and ritualistic practice. The need to practice using up-to-date evidence is a requirement of many professionals and is expressed for nurses in the Nurses' Code of Professional Conduct (Nursing and Midwifery Council 2008). These practitioners cannot afford to perpetuate traditional and ritualistic practice if it is at the expense of developments that are beneficial to the patient and the profession. Professionals are accountable for their practice and must be able to ensure that the best possible care is being made available so that practice can be justified as the most appropriate.

INTUITION AND TACIT KNOWLEDGE

The use of intuition and tacit knowledge is apparent in health and social care practice, but cannot easily be explained. For example, the physiotherapist who knows what the patient's needs are without detailed assessment, the nurse who knows when a patient's life is at an end but cannot explain why this is known, uses intuitive and tacit knowledge. Intuition was described some time ago as perhaps having acute sensitivity, a sixth sense (Burnard, 1989), built on knowledge and experience, which is applied to decision-making and problem solving. Tacit knowledge is developed through the experience accumulated from practice over a period of time. It is the development of 'expert opinion' that is a synthesis of formal knowledge and clinical expertise. It is suggested that much of this knowledge is passed on to future generations of practitioners through modelling of actions, tasks and attitudes (Gunilla et al., 2002).

The lack of objectivity and ability to identify a rationale behind intuitive and tacit decisions has affected the recognition of this source of knowledge, preventing it being viewed as a valid **phenomenon** for scientific investigation. Yet, it is argued that there are many situations where the application of intuitive and tacit knowledge is essential. These include ethical dilemmas where, for example, the possible response or reaction is unknown and professionals will draw on intuitive knowledge to inform practice. As the debates surrounding the use of tacit and intuitive knowledge in nursing practice continue (Gunilla et al., 2002; Whitehead, 2005), there needs to be a recognition that these forms of knowledge can inform the development of personal knowledge. Such knowledge might therefore form part of the understanding that informs professional practice.

Personal knowledge is individual and is developed through experience in practice events and situations. The experienced health and social care professional brings additional sensitivity into prac-tice. This use of intuition and tacit knowledge enables the delivery of the best possible care. Within nursing, Benner (1984) sees the experienced nurse as the expert clinician who uses intuition and tacit knowledge as part of delivering holistic (total) care to the patient. Benner (1984) suggests that 'know how' knowledge, which highlights the difference between the beginner or novice and the expert practitioner, should be valued more highly. The develop-ment of 'knowledge that' into 'knowledge how' as part of acquiring intuition allows the expert practitioner to view the complete situa-tion and therefore apply holistic care, using past experience and knowledge. The value of intuition to holistic care is discussed by Agan (1987) who links intuitive knowledge to the development of personal knowledge through **reflective practice**.

Problem-solving through reflective practice was popularised by Argyris and Schön (1974), with the later work of Schön (1987) sug-gesting the development of two types of reflective skill. Reflection-in-action, where the practitioner is appraising care and making changes at the time, is compared with reflection-on-action, which follows the event and uses an analysis of preceding practice to shape the future.

The work of Schön (1987) has been influential in health and social care practice and education. Though the work has been criti-cised (Greenwood, 1993), the value given to reflective practice in building personal knowledge, and ultimately in developing intui-tion and tacit knowledge, confirms the place of such knowledge in supporting health and social care practice.

COMMON SENSE

To use the words 'common sense' is to suggest that something is widely accepted or generally known, as well as being logically rea-soned and thought through. Sensible people would usually apply common sense. Knowledge based on common sense is therefore gained through accepted understanding, developed through indi-vidual experience that is not associated with any formal education or training.

Its value as a source of health and social care knowledge on which to base care is limited, as can be seen through the examina-tion of a common sense approach to certain clinical practices. Common sense might lead to covering a warm but shivering child with extra blankets. Learned knowledge of the need to reduce a child's temperature and therefore the shivering will result in the removal of any extra blankets and clothing. People often refer to childcare generally as common sense. The ability of parents to 'bring up' children will be evaluated on the basis of the amount of common sense the parents are thought to have. 'Mr and Mrs Smith will be "good" parents because they have a lot of common sense.' While it may be true that Mr and Mrs Smith will be 'good' parents, there is nothing that is at all common about the approach to parenthood. This can be seen in the plethora of texts available for parents that offer differing advice on all aspects of childcare.

As common sense is derived from individual experience, it is naturally limited, can be **biased**, and is drawn from individual reasoning rather than from external sources. The rationale for practice is consequently unsupported and may lead to the delivery of care that is not the best available, or the most appropriate.

Challenging practice based on common sense can be fraught with problems, as for the individual the practice is reasonable and understandable, and to them it makes 'common' sense. Questioning common sense is, however, necessary to ensure care is of a high standard, and to prevent the perpetuation of practices that are restricted by individual experience and bias.

Common sense can provide a useful approach to care delivery, but health and social care professionals, as accountable practitioners, must critically examine and evaluate practice, choosing a knowledge base which supports professional and quality care.

TRIAL AND ERROR

Most of us use trial and error in solving problems on a day-to-day basis. When presented with a problem we will try one way of resolving it, and if this fails, different approaches will be taken until a solution is found. The solution is then remembered and used if the same or a similar problem occurs again.

Trial and error will only provide a solution to one specific problem and is therefore limited in its use. It is, however, an important source of knowledge, as others may recommend solutions for use when faced with similar problems. For example, much advice is offered to people with common colds, such as to take high doses of vitamin C, and stay in the warm. The implications of passing on knowledge gained through trial and error learning may be to contribute to traditional knowledge or in fact to authoritative knowledge that is considered later. Knowledge based on trial and error, which may ultimately be developed into traditional or authoritative knowledge, can provide a valid basis for care.

AUTHORITY

Knowledge originating from people in positions of authority, who are often perceived as experts, can be accepted as a reasonable basis for practice. There are many individuals who impart authoritative knowledge: specialist practitioners, senior managers, lecturers, medical staff, therapists. In fact all personnel in the health and social care environments have the potential to be seen as an authority. This may develop from the person's position, which is likely to be one of power, or the person's perceived knowledge and experience, or the very personality and self-portrayal of the individual.

As a source of knowledge, the expert may have much to offer that will benefit students, staff, and ultimately patients. There is, however, a concern that the expert will not be challenged, that the position of authority is above reproach and that the knowledge of the expert can be used without questioning the source. It is possible for the expert to offer a vehicle for the perpetuation of traditional and ritualistic practice, of practices which support the expert's preferences and idiosyncrasies, rather than practice which is in fact sound and based on fact. There are many examples of such practice. The teaching of cardio-pulmonary resuscitation has varied according to the individual demonstrating basic life support skills, and continues to vary despite the development of Resuscitation Council (UK) Guidelines (2010) that are based on the current evidence base. It is therefore important for the recipient of authoritative knowledge to establish the original source of the information and determine a basis for practice that is justifiable.

It should also be remembered that experts impart knowledge through publication. The content of any journal article or text should not be accepted as true just because it is published, but it should be questioned and critically appraised. All health and social care professionals need critical reading skills to determine the strengths and weaknesses of published work, and should be encouraged to adopt a questioning approach (see Chapter 11).

Policies and procedures are also used to guide practice. Many procedures used in the past gave step-by-step instructions for the practitioner to follow. More recently, the procedural approach has been succeeded by sound principles. These are less prescriptive and offer guidelines for safe practice. It is, however, important that the knowledge behind clinical principles is established. Rationales should be offered, which include referenced facts and high-quality evidence.

SCIENTIFIC KNOWLEDGE

Scientific knowledge is seen as informing health and social care practice through solving problems in a logical, systematic and rigorous way. Scientific knowledge generated through research activity uses a rigorous approach to obtain findings used to inform practice (Moule and Goodman, 2014). Chapter 1 presented definitions of research, all of which suggest a systematic approach to testing and generating knowledge. This suggests that the research process, described in Chapter 3, is used to provide a logical and systematic structure to problem-solving.

The need for scientific knowledge is acknowledged in the opening chapter, as is the need for education and training to enable health and social care practitioners to develop research awareness skills. Such skills are necessary to critically analyse and appraise research, thus allowing the identification of strengths and weaknesses in the research process (see Chapter 11).

The need for the health and social care professions to develop a scientific knowledge base for practice is also established, with research being viewed as a professional necessity. It is vital that the accountable practitioner can confidently deliver care based on reliable research evidence. There are benefits for the patient and professionals in developing research-based health and social care practice.

The development of scientific knowledge in health and social care has its difficulties and limitations. Just as health and social care professionals need to be critical in their appraisal of other **sources of knowledge**, so they need to be critical of research. The strengths and weaknesses of scientific knowledge must be identified through **critical appraisal**, as is highlighted in Chapter 11.

One independent organisation supporting practitioners in the development of evidence-based practice is the National Institute for Health and Care Excellence (NICE). NICE is responsible for providing national guidelines on the promotion of good health and the prevention and treatment of ill health. NICE provides guidance in conditions and disease, public health, treatments, procedures and devices (see www.nice.org.uk).

All research is fallible, all will have both strengths and limitations that should be considered when evaluating any of the recommendations made for practice.

The very nature of health and social care practice causes research difficulties, including ethical problems and measurement issues. Certain research may not gain ethical approval. For example, delaying mobilisation of patients following admission to hospital ignores current best practice recommendations issued by the previous National Institute for Clinical Excellence, now National Institute for Health and Care Excellence (NICE, 2010a) and could endanger participants. Such research would be seen as negligent and unethical.

Though there are many measurement tools available to the researcher (see Chapter 9), the collection of high-quality information, as part of a qualitative approach, poses difficulties. The measurement of, for example, opinions, feelings, thoughts, viewpoint, behaviour, can challenge research.

Additional difficulties lie in health and social care itself. The impetus for research can be uncertain, the education and research skills of the professions are still developing, and the application of research knowledge to practice is not always uniform.

Health and social care professionals need to acquire research knowledge and skills, to shape the future of professional research. These skills are now developed to a basic level within all pre-registration courses, which often require the completion of a research critique, research project or dissertation. Most post-registration courses include research awareness skills and there are specialised research courses at master's level, and increasing opportunities for doctoral-level studies. Career pathways are developing for those professionals who choose to make a career in research and practice or education. The UK Clinical Research Collaboration (UKCRC) established in 2004 has the aim of increasing research capacity across the NHS workforce. Following a consultation process (UKCRC, 2006), new clinical research career structures for nurses, midwives and allied health professionals have been developed in different ways across the UK. In England, the Clinical Academic Training Programme for nurses, midwives and allied health professionals will include four integrated levels of research training, consisting of masters, doctorate, clinical lectureship and senior academic clinical lectureship.

Scientific knowledge may not always be the most appropriate source of information on which to base practice, but the use of scientific enquiry can establish the basis for care. It should be remembered that all types of knowledge discussed in this chapter can provide a basis for health and social care practice and the type of knowledge base employed may change with time and context as there is no single permanent truth.

KEY POINTS

- Health and social care professionals need to be aware of the concept of evidence-based practice.
- The development of health and social care theory has been multi-dimensional, with knowledge being generated from many sources.
- Research must support measurement and the testing of knowledge in a systematic way.
- The professions are still developing research skills and expertise.

FURTHER READING

Benner, P., Tanner, C. and Chesla, C. (2009). *Expertise in nursing practice: Caring, clinical judgement and ethics* (2nd edn). New York: Springer.
Rolfe, G. (1998). *Expanding nursing knowledge* (2nd edn). Oxford: Butterworth Heinemann.

WEBSITES

National Institute for Health and Care Excellence: www.nice.org.uk
Nursing and Midwifery Council: www.nmc-uk.org
Resuscitation Council: www.resus.org.uk
UK Clinical Research Collaboration: www.ukcrc.org.uk

3 OVERVIEW OF THE RESEARCH PROCESS

LEARNING OUTCOMES

On completion of this chapter the reader should be able to:

- identify the stages of the research process
- understand the interrelationships between the stages of the research process
- appreciate how the research process guides research activity.

KEY CONCEPTS

- research process
- qualitative approach
- quantitative approach

INTRODUCTION

This chapter offers a broad overview of the stages that comprise the research process, discusses the functions of the different processes, and highlights their use as a framework for research activity. In doing so, the chapter provides the basis for many of the following chapters, where issues raised will be further explored.

The research process is a framework, which enables researchers to start with a research problem and follow a series of logical stages, to end with an outcome or result (see Figure 3.1). It is a theoretical model which, when applied by researchers, may not be followed in a sequential way. It is more likely that stages of the process will run concurrently, interrelate and interchange, and some may be completely omitted. For example, the **research questions** may be formulated initially and then redefined or completely rewritten as the researcher has an opportunity to reflect on the progress of the research study.

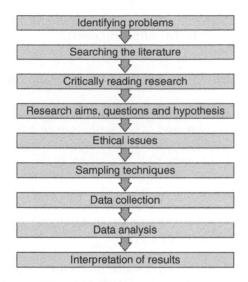

Figure 3.1   *Stages of the research process*

In undertaking a research study, the researcher's progression through the research process will depend on the research approach taken, which can be qualitative or quantitative. The outcomes of qualitative approaches are achieved without the use of statistical measures, although some do include a degree of statistical analysis (see Chapter 6). In contrast, the quantitative approach relies on statistical measures for its results and therefore necessitates the use of larger **samples** and more structured data collection tools (Moule and Goodman, 2014).

Reflection by the researcher at each stage of the research process can be considered beneficial to the ultimate outcomes of the research. At each stage of the research process the researcher may make alterations to the continuation of the study based on progressive evaluations and thus hope to improve the final outcome and results.

Many writers, such as Bell (2010), consider the research process from an operational perspective. They discuss how to use the research process to write a research proposal (a plan of proposed work completed by a researcher prior to undertaking research). In particular, they describe how to plan and carry out a research project, and finally consider how to present the research findings.

For most health and social care professionals the research process provides a basis for evaluating and appraising completed research in a critical way, as is further discussed in Chapter 11. Knowledge of the stages of the research process therefore enables practitioners to read research reports. This is facilitated as researchers use the research process to structure the written presentation of research findings in reports and journal articles (see www.journalofadvancednursing.com).

INVOLVEMENT OF THE PUBLIC IN THE RESEARCH PROCESS

In recent years **patient and public involvement** (PPI) in health care research has increased. The public are involved in a more comprehensive way, with research being undertaken with and by patients, rather than being done for, or about the public (Involve, 2012). This approach recognises the important of involving patients and the public in all stages of the research process, so that they can influence research questions and design. Whilst the level of involvement varies across projects, patient and public input can be manifest in a number of ways:

1. identifying and prioritising research problems
2. informing the development of the design
3. involvement in the development of materials for ethics approval such as consent forms
4. design of data collection tools
5. advising on, and supporting recruitment
6. involvement in data analysis
7. involvement in the dissemination of research findings.

IDENTIFYING PROBLEMS

The first stage in the research process is to define a problem. Health and social care professionals experiencing or observing a particular issue in their practice may generate the research problem at a local level. Research problems may also result from the identification of research priorities by, for example, the Department of Health, which funds specific research studies into practice concerns, such as cancer, stroke care or mental health. Charitable or private organisations such as Help the Aged, Joseph Rowntree Foundation, Mental Health Foundation and pharmaceutical companies also fund research. Service users and carers can also make a valuable contribution to identifying research problems and issues.

The researcher can be considering research problems that pertain to local, national, European or international issues, and is likely to be working as part of a research team. Whatever the scale of the research, the researcher must be clear about the relevance of researching the identified problem and have a clear understanding of the purpose of the research. In other words, what problem is the research trying to address, what is the research trying to achieve, what are the outcomes hoping to show, and how will the outcomes be used?

Whatever the purpose of the research, the research problem needs to be researchable. The researcher needs to consider how the problem can be investigated, what type of results are likely to be generated and how they would be analysed. In addition, the researcher needs to address any ethical issues, such as whether service users or staff are involved in the investigation.

The research problem is often broad and requires some refinement to form the research aims, questions and **hypothesis** (see later discussions and Chapter 7). This is achieved by further exploration of the problem area, which includes searching and reviewing relevant literature.

SEARCHING THE LITERATURE

Having identified the research issue, the researcher must undertake a **literature search** before refining the problem. The literature search involves the retrieval of literature that is relevant to the research problem. The literature search should continue throughout the period of the research study to include any relevant literature published during the study period. However, the main literature search is likely to take place in the early stages of the research process.

The approach taken to searching the literature is important as this affects the breadth and depth of literature obtained. Different lines of enquiry may tempt the researcher as the search continues. The researcher must avoid diversions that have no relevance to the study. The literature search needs to be structured around key areas, perhaps starting with key concepts or words, and should progress systematically with the original research problem providing the continued focus for the search.

There are many aids to searching literature available, which are fully discussed in Chapter 5. It is important that the researcher has sufficient knowledge and skills to access the resources. In addition, the researcher should use a reference or database system, recording details of literature that has been obtained, or is likely to be accessed during the study. These records will be used throughout the study and may be of use in the future, particularly if further research is undertaken.

As well as researchers, all health and social care professionals need to be able to undertake a literature search. Literature-searching skills are important for professionals. Such skills will facilitate the development of practice, supporting the acquisition and updating of knowledge. This is essential for the development of **evidence-based practice**, and ultimately the quality of care. Professionals undertaking further courses will also need to use literature-searching skills to meet coursework requirements.

CRITICALLY READING RESEARCH

The reading of research literature often occurs concurrently with the literature search; however, the two stages are discussed separately to highlight fundamental differences between the two. The review of the research literature requires the use of **critical appraisal** skills to determine the strengths and weaknesses of the research, whereas the literature search is used to identify the literature for review.

The process of critical review requires knowledge of the research process and can be assisted by the use of a framework outlining the stages of critical appraisal (see Appendix 3). Critical reading skills used in the process of critical appraisal are discussed in Chapter 11. These skills are essential to the researcher and of importance to all health and social care professionals. If practice is to be developed from an objective research base, professionals must have the skills needed to analyse literature and offer an objective appraisal of research findings.

In reviewing the literature critically, the researcher may obtain the answer to the research problem, thus negating the need for further research. Alternatively, the need for further research may be confirmed, and suggestions as to how the study should progress may be gained. For example, the research methodology could be replicated, or the data collection tool, such as a **questionnaire**, could, with the permission of the original researchers, be reproduced for use in the study.

RESEARCH AIMS, QUESTIONS AND HYPOTHESIS

The research aims, questions and hypothesis give focus and direction to the research study. The research aim, or aims, are generated, outlining what the research study is hoping to achieve. The research question is developed following the **literature review**, and narrows the original problem into a more concise statement.

The research hypothesis gives even greater focus to the research, as it offers a prediction of the anticipated research outcomes. The hypothesis is a statement that is tested by the researcher and, dependent on the findings, will either be accepted as true or rejected. Fuller explanations of this are given in Chapter 7.

The researchers need to ensure they address the research aims, questions and hypotheses within the study.

ETHICAL ISSUES

All researchers need to work ethically, adhering to ethical principles that seek to protect vulnerable participants. Ethical issues permeate all stages of the research process, including the decision to undertake the research, the research design and its execution. Key ethical principles are discussed in Chapter 4, along with ways of working ethically and the processes of ethical governance in health and social care.

SAMPLING TECHNIQUES

Sampling involves the collection of information on which decisions can be made and from which conclusions can be drawn. The selection of a sample is therefore a very important part of the research process. Before a sample is selected the researcher identifies the target population, which includes the entire membership of the group in which the researcher is interested and from which information can be collected.

The **target population** could include participants or incidents. For example, the researcher may be interested in obtaining information from community physiotherapists. All community physiotherapists would therefore form the target population.

It is unlikely that the researcher would collect information from the entire target population, but a sample would be selected to take part in the study. The most important feature of sampling is the degree to which the sample represents the target population. For the sample to be truly representative, the participants need to reflect the target population in as many ways as possible. If the target population is student radiographers following the diagnostic radiography programme, the sample needs to be made up of students studying diagnostic rather than therapeutic radiography. Limitation of difference between the target population and sample is achieved to some degree through the use of accepted sampling techniques.

Sampling techniques fall into two sampling strategies, **probability** and **non-probability sampling**. Probability sampling involves the use of random selection, with every member of the target population having an equal chance of being included in the sample. There are different probability sampling techniques, including simple, stratified, systematic and cluster sampling. Non-probability samples are selected without the use of random selection. The inclusion of subjects can be through convenience, quota, purposive and snowball sampling techniques. The different sampling techniques are discussed in Chapter 8.

RESEARCH DESIGN

The research design is a plan of how the research will proceed. It includes consideration of the proposed research approach, and the research methods, data collection tools, and the methods of **data analysis** that are to be employed.

The research design might use quantitative or qualitative approaches to the research (see Chapter 6). This will be reflected in the sample size used, data collection method and techniques employed, and will be most evident in the results obtained and their analysis.

A **pilot study** is used as part of the research design, often to check sampling techniques, to test the **validity** and **reliability** of data collection tools. It also gives the researcher an opportunity to practise research skills, such as interviewing techniques.

The researcher will reflect on the experiences gained during the pilot study to refine aspects of the main study. This can provide financial benefits, and facilitate the effective use of resources in the final research study.

DATA COLLECTION TECHNIQUES

The researcher's choice of data collection instrument is influenced by the research approach taken. For example, a quantitative approach may use structured data collection techniques, such as a questionnaire; whereas a qualitative approach may include the use of unstructured **interviews** or observational techniques.

The most commonly used data collection techniques include physiological and psychological measures, measuring scales, **questionnaires**, interviews, **observations** and documentary evidence (see Chapter 9).

DATA ANALYSIS

The method of data analysis used will depend on the research approach taken and the techniques of data collection employed. To aid analysis, the results, often described as **raw data**, will be processed in some way.

Raw data generated through quantitative approaches tends to be numerical. Analysis of numerical data is often achieved using computer packages. Statistical tests are applied to the raw data to generate statistical results that are interpreted by the researcher (see Chapter 10).

Research that follows qualitative approaches generates data such as text, which is not amenable to statistical analysis. It is the content of the text that is important. The analysis may begin during the stage of data collection, and the researcher can begin to identify trends or themes while gathering information.

INTERPRETATION OF RESULTS

This stage of the research process includes both interpretation of the results and the formulation of conclusions. Interpretation of the findings occurs in the light of the original research aims, questions and any hypothesis statements made, while reflecting on previous research studies identified in the critical review of the literature.

Discussions should highlight the researcher's interpretation of the results, acknowledge any limitations of the research process and consider the **generalisability** of the results (whether the results from the sample can be applied to a target population). The relevance and significance that the research findings might have for practice and further research would also be inferred from the research findings. For example, a change in existing practice may be recommended, or suggestions for further research may be made.

PRESENTATION AND DISSEMINATION

This final stage of the research process concentrates on the communication of the research findings to any sponsors or funding body and members of the health and social care professions, as well as to any participants, such as patients and clients. The research process is often used as a framework for presentation. **Dissemination** activity can occur at local, national and international levels. A research dissertation can be made available through a local trust or university library. Research findings can be presented through posters or presentations at local research clubs and interest groups. Wider communication of the results can also be achieved through publication in national or international journals and the presentation of papers at a range of conferences. Internet web pages and electronic media, such as electronic mail, social media sites and discussion groups, can also provide a forum for dissemination.

Researchers hope that the research findings will increase the body of health and social care knowledge, and contribute to the improvement of practice. Further discussions on the dissemination of research are included in Chapter 12.

KEY POINTS

- The research process is a framework that enables researchers to start with a problem and follow a series of logical and sequential steps, to end with an outcome or result.
- The research process includes the following stages: identifying the problems, searching the literature, critically reading research, setting research aims, questions and hypothesis, ethical issues, sampling techniques, data collection, data analysis and interpretation of results.
- Patients and the public are increasingly involved in all stages of the research process.
- Research problems can be generated locally or identified as research priorities by research funders, such as the government or charitable organisations.
- Understanding the stages of the research process enables health and social care professionals to identify and read research studies.

FURTHER READING

Alston, M. and Bowles, W. (2012). *Research for social workers: An introduction to methods* (3rd edn). London: Routledge.

Bowling, A. (2009). *Research methods in health: Investigating health and health services* (3rd edn). Buckingham: Open University Press.
Hicks, C. (2009). *Research methods for clinical therapists* (5th edn). Edinburgh: Churchill Livingstone.
Moule, P. and Goodman, M. (2014). *Nursing research: An introduction* (2nd edn). London: Sage.
Polit, D. and Beck, C. (2014). *Essentials of nursing research: Appraising evidence for nursing practice* (8th edn). Philadelphia, PA: Lippincott Williams and Wilkins.
Robson, C. (2011). *Real world research: A resource for social scientists and practitioner-researchers* (3rd edn). Oxford: Blackwell.

WEBSITE

Journal of Advanced Nursing: www.journalofadvancednursing.com

4 ETHICAL ISSUES

INTRODUCTION

More and more health and social care practitioners are becoming involved in practice-based research. Some are undertaking research projects as part of course work, and some health and social care practitioners work as research nurses, research physiotherapists, research fellows in social services, or as members of a multidisciplinary research team. However, there are many more practitioners who are less directly involved in the whole process, perhaps through collecting data from patients and clients, such as administering client satisfaction **questionnaires**, collecting urine or blood samples, or gathering information for other research workers. Other people undertaking research could be social scientists, psychologists, health service researchers, and doctors. Whether a health and social care practitioner is the project leader, or a sole researcher, or collecting data for someone else, there are responsibilities with regard to the ethics and governance of research on humans. At all stages of the research process there are ethical implications, including the decision to undertake research or not, and the issue of undertaking poorly designed or executed research. Health and social care practitioners need to be aware of these issues in their own place of work.

ETHICAL PRINCIPLES

Ethical principles distinguish socially acceptable behaviour from that which is considered socially unacceptable. There are a number of 'codes of conduct' or sets of principles and guidelines produced by professional and disciplinary bodies, both nationally and internationally, such as the British Psychological Society, the British Sociological Association, the International Council of Nurses, the Royal College of Nursing, the Joint University Council Social Work Education Committee and the General Medical Council. They all draw on the Declaration of Geneva, the Nuremberg Code and the Declaration of Helsinki: ethical guidelines produced as a result of human experimentation undertaken mainly during the Second World War. These build on basic human rights, now almost universally acknowledged.

The key ethical principles and basic human rights that should be followed throughout a research study in order to protect clients and patients are identified in Table 4.1.

These principles and rights can be used as a framework to appraise research designs and methods and to examine the effects of research on the participants. It must be noted that some research designs will need to be considered in certain and more specific ways. For example, in some ethnographic studies, the participants may not know they are being observed and therefore have no choice about participating or not; in disseminating the research findings of **action research**, issues of **confidentiality** may be more difficult; in experimental research a random selection might result in a voluntary group who do not represent the **target population**, being better educated, of a higher social class or more socially involved.

Table 4.1   *Ethical principles and human rights in research*

The principle of veracity:

- Telling the truth, being honest and being sincere.
- The right of participants to have full disclosure before participating in research.

The principle of justice:

- Being fair to participants and not giving preference to some over others.
- Participants' needs must come before the objectives of the study.
- A duty to avoid discrimination, abuse or exploitation of the participants on the grounds of race, religion, sex, age, class or sexual orientation.

The principle of beneficence (or non-maleficence):

- The research should benefit both the individual participants, and society in general.
- A duty to do good and prevent harm (physical, psychological, social and economic).
- A duty of care to protect the weak and vulnerable.
- Defence of the weak, vulnerable or incompetent (advocacy role).

The principle of fidelity and respect:

- The building of trust where the researcher is obliged to safeguard the welfare of participants.
- A duty to respect the rights, autonomy and dignity of participants.
- A duty to promote the well-being and autonomy of participants.
- The right to self-determination (the freedom to decide whether to participate or not, and to withdraw at any time).
- The right to privacy and respect.
- The right to anonymity and confidentiality.

In addition to the methods and procedures used in research, the subject matter can also cause ethical concern, such as in the area of abuse or criminal activity, or with particularly vulnerable groups, such as the very old, or people with a severe learning disability or severe mental illness, or the dying. The challenge for readers of research, or those undertaking research in some way, is to maintain a balance between rigour and respect so that research evidence is produced ethically.

INFORMED CONSENT

Informed consent is a **concept** familiar to many health and social care practitioners, particularly with reference to treatment and care. The principle of informed consent is also applied to patients and clients who are potential research participants and it is the fundamental ethical principle involved in research. There are a number of important considerations when research involves human volunteers, some of which have been discussed earlier: participants should know that they are taking part in research; they should give written informed consent to take part in the study; and they should be assured that they can withdraw at any time during the study. As part of providing information prior to participants giving consent, the researcher should explain how and why participants were selected, and who is undertaking and financing the study. Written information might also include: an explanation of how long the study will take; whether there will be any discomfort; whether there are any conceivable risks or costs such as psychological or emotional distress resulting from self-disclosure; whether there may be any loss of privacy; and if there might be any loss of time, or monetary costs associated with participating in the research. Likewise, participants should be informed of any potential benefits, such as material gains or comfort in being able to discuss their situation or escape from normal routine; knowledge that they may be helping others; and possibly enhanced self-esteem as a result of receiving special attention. Participants should also be given information about who to contact if they have any questions or complaints relating to the research. Written information should be given to the potential participants, and where possible they should be given time to consider whether they want to take part before seeking their written informed consent. Participants should have the power of free choice so that they are able to voluntarily consent or decline to participate in the research. Any researcher undertaking research with NHS patients can access clear guidance on the preparation of written information from the National Research Ethics Service (NRES) (www.nres.nhs.uk).

PRACTICE EXAMPLE

When reading a research paper the process of gaining informed consent can be presented as part of the methodology or in a separate section related to ethical issues. The amount of detail provided can vary, though the key processes involved should be included, as in the following example from Rønnevig et al. (2009). Their research investigated

(Continued)

(Continued)

patients' experiences of living with irritable bowel syndrome and involved collecting data from 13 participants through qualitative interviews. The informed consent process included:

- securing ethics committee approval
- provision of written information to participants
- written assurance that confidentiality will be maintained
- written assurance that the participants could withdraw at any time without providing a reason
- written consent.

The paper also talks about obtaining Data Protection Committee approval required in the local setting. Any participant wishing to withdraw in this example should also be able to do so without prejudice. In some cases it may not be possible to ensure confidentiality, for example when collecting data from a very specific and easily identifiable group of people. In such cases the researcher should report that participants were informed that confidentiality could not be assured. The researcher should also report any other steps taken to support confidentiality, such as allowing the participants to comment on quotes or analysis in the content of a report or paper prior to wider dissemination.

VULNERABLE PARTICIPANTS

Some people are considered to be vulnerable. They may be competent to give consent to participate, but may find it difficult to withhold consent if they are put under implicit or explicit pressure. People with learning disabilities, or who have a mental health problem, or are frail and elderly, or are living in an institution, may all be considered vulnerable, as may children and young people, and women who are pregnant. They may be vulnerable because of hidden pressures or the risk of unintended side effects. Including vulnerable people in research requires careful consideration, as to exclude such groups from research may be a form of discrimination. Therefore, researchers need to justify why certain groups of people should be included in research, and consider not just the individual's ability to comprehend the information given, but – just as importantly – the form and nature of the explanation given and the way that consent is obtained, particularly if participants are only intermittently competent to consent or have difficulty retaining information.

Some adults may not be competent to give consent. There must be clear justification for researchers including these groups of participants in research and it should never be undertaken if it could be completed equally well with other adults. If a researcher wants to involve adults who are unable to give consent, it should be limited to the areas of research related to their incapacity. A researcher will also need to demonstrate that the research could be of direct benefit to, or improve knowledge of, their health or the health of people with the same state of health or same incapacity. The researcher must also establish that the individual has not expressed any objection either verbally or physically and that participation will not cause the participants emotional, physical or psychological harm.

Researchers may want to involve children and young people in research. However, as a potentially vulnerable group, they must not be exploited and may be unable to express their own needs, protect themselves from harm or make informed choices about being involved in research. If children and young people are not competent to independently give consent to participate in research, the consent of someone with parental responsibility must be obtained.

Researchers can undertake research with vulnerable participants or those who lack capacity to give consent provided the requirements of the Mental Capacity Act 2005 are fulfilled. The Act sets out duties to ensure that individuals who lack capacity are treated with respect and their rights are protected. The need for the research must be justified and it must be clear that the research cannot be carried out on individuals with the capacity to consent.

Health and social care practitioners must be fully aware of the issues surrounding informed consent. Guidance on gaining informed consent from patients and service users in the NHS and example forms can be found on the NRES website. If a health and social care practitioner feels that a client or patient does not fully understand their role as a research participant, they have a responsibility to make this known to the researcher. Likewise, if the practitioner feels that a patient or client wishes to withdraw from a study, or that the research is having an adverse effect on the participants, they have a responsibility to make this known to an appropriate person in authority.

PRACTICE EXAMPLE

Cameron and Murphy (2006) discuss the issues of including people with learning and communication disabilities in research. The project received ethical approval from the NHS Ethics of Research Committee and the University Ethics Committee. A total of 48 participants were recruited to the study, divided into one of four groups according to their ability to understand information-carrying words. The methods of recruitment used highlight ways of overcoming some of the issues of working with vulnerable adults discussed previously. For example, there were key strategic approaches used in recruitment, obtaining consent and continuing consent:

- Recruitment included the use of a letter and information sheet sent to speech and language therapists working with adults with learning disabilities. The therapists were able to explain the study to the potential participants. The letter used accessible language principles to aid understanding.
- Consent was gained through an appointment process involving the potential participant and their carer. The researcher explained the research, again using spoken and visual communication. They repeated explanations, gave time in between explanations, explained the project in stages, used visual aids, short and simple sentences, allowed the potential participant to read, look at and inspect information. The carer acted as an observer and confirmed the participant's decision either to take part or decline. The participants were able to either sign or make a mark of consent at the end on a form that used short written sentences and symbols.
- Ongoing consent was gained at each stage of data collection. This involved a telephone call prior to each of the four face-to-face interviews to confirm continuing consent. At the start of each interview, consent was reiterated.

The principles of providing visual and brief written information are good practice when working with people with learning and communication difficulties but could also be used in consent processes for other research groups.

CONFIDENTIALITY AND ANONYMITY

Participants in research have a right to expect that any information they provide will be treated confidentially and that information about them will only be disclosed with their consent. There must be a clear understanding between the researcher and participant concerning the use to be made of the data provided, and how personal information will be stored.

Anonymity can be maintained by not using the names and addresses of participants, and assigning an identity number or code. The code to the names should be kept separately and securely so that the researcher cannot link data with a particular participant. The research participants should not be discussed beyond the needs of the project team, and the data must be kept secure at all times. This is particularly important with data stored on a computer. Access to the data should be restricted to those people who have a legitimate reason to see it.

If confidentiality or anonymity cannot be guaranteed, participants must be warned in advance before they agree to participate. For example, maintaining anonymity when studying a specialised grouping of say the social care workforce could be problematic. In these cases the researchers can ensure the participants review the presentation of findings, agreeing verbatim quotes used, before wider **dissemination** in the form of a report or journal paper. Confidentiality is a principle of research that is found in all professional codes and guidelines. If information needs to be disclosed in the public interest without a participant's consent, there must be a benefit to the individual or society that outweighs the individual's right to confidentiality. Researchers need to abide by the requirements of the law, including the Data Protection Act 1998, Human Rights Act 1998, the Health and Social Care Act 2001, Human Tissue Act 2004, the Mental Capacity Act 2005 and the Public Interest Disclosure Act 1998, which defines a public disclosure as where in good faith an employee reasonably believes:

- a criminal offence has been committed, is being committed, or is likely to be committed
- a person has failed, is failing, or is likely to fail to comply with any legal obligation to which they are subject
- a miscarriage of justice has occurred, is occurring or is likely to occur
- the health or safety of an individual has been, is being, or is likely to be endangered
- the environment has been, is being, or is likely to be damaged
- information related to any of the above has been, is being or is likely to be deliberately concealed.

Decisions about breaking confidentiality 'in the public interest' are complex, with each case being considered on its merits as to whether the duty of confidence to the research participant should prevail over the disclosure of information.

THE HEALTH AND SOCIAL CARE PRACTITIONER AS DATA COLLECTOR

Health and social care practitioners collecting data for research purposes must be as meticulous, accurate and reliable as they would be in collecting data in their normal work. There could be a conflict when a health and social care practitioner takes on a 'dual role' as practitioner and researcher. Practitioners working in this dual role must ensure that the data collected for research purposes is kept separate from patient information gathered in the daily work unless the research participant's consent is obtained. Practitioners must also be satisfied that any 'funded' research is ethically and scientifically sound and that, as individuals, they are not associated with any promotion of a particular product.

Health and social care practitioners must always uphold the principles of their own codes of conduct. They should possess the relevant research skills and knowledge compatible with the demands of the proposed research and acknowledge any limitations of their ability. As highlighted in an earlier chapter, a health and social care practitioner who is undertaking research must be certain that the knowledge sought is not already available.

RESEARCH ETHICS COMMITTEES

Before researchers start their research project, they need to seek an independent ethical review of their proposed research. There are formalised procedures for researchers seeking ethical approval for research which involves clients and patients; access to notes and records; access to staff within health and social services; and access to premises within health and social care. In the case of health research, an NHS **Research Ethics Committee** will scrutinise research applications and give opinions as to whether the proposed research has considered all ethical issues. Social services departments may also use an NHS Research Ethics Committee, a University Ethics Committee or their own committee in order to seek an independent ethical review of any proposed research which falls into their sphere of responsibility. Applications to Research Ethics Committee are standardised and submitted through the Integrated Research Application System (IRAS).

Ethics committees are likely to follow the principles outlined earlier in this chapter in order to review potential research projects. Membership of the committee is multi-professional, with members having experience across all types of research design. Laypeople are likely to be members, and they will be able to give the perspective of an ordinary individual who is not in professional practice. Ethical review involves an application form, a research protocol that provides details of the proposed research, copies of the research instruments (for example, questionnaires, interview schedules) and most importantly participant information sheets and consent forms. Some committees require the researchers to attend a committee meeting to answer questions about the proposed work, and a researcher may not commence their research until the Research Ethics Committee has given a favourable opinion.

RESEARCH GOVERNANCE

In addition to gaining a favourable opinion following an independent ethical review, researchers conducting research in health and social services need to have their research approved by the NHS Trust(s) or social service department(s) where they wish to conduct their research. This requires them to satisfy the NHS Trust/social service department that the research has fulfilled a number of **research governance** requirements. These are:

- high scientific quality
- peer review
- identified sponsor (usually the employer of the lead researcher)
- financial probity
- adequate monitoring
- involvement of users of the research
- sufficient indemnity and compensation
- evidence of independent ethical review.

Research governance has come about as a result of a number of high-profile research scandals and increasing public awareness of ethical issues.

KEY POINTS

- Health and social care practitioners must be aware of ethical issues when they are reading research.
- Informed consent is an important consideration in all research involving human participants.
- Some research participants, such as children and people with a mental health problem, are considered vulnerable.
- Confidentiality and anonymity should be maintained.
- Research Ethics Committees and research governance procedures serve the interests of patients with regard to research.

FURTHER READING

Department of Health (2008). *Research governance framework for health and social care* (2nd edn). London: Department of Health.

Fontela, M. and Rycroft-Malone, J. (2006). Research governance and ethics: a resource for novice researchers. *Nursing Standard*, 20 (23), 41–6.

Royal College of Nursing (2009). *Research ethics: RCN guidance for nurses*. London: RCN.

WEBSITES

Government Legislation: www.legislation.gov.uk

International Council of Nurses: www.icn.ch

National Research Ethics Service: www.nres.npsa.nhs.uk

Royal College of nursing: www.rcn.org.uk

Joint University Committee, Social Work Education Committee: Research Ethics: www.juc.ac.uk/swec-research-code.html

5 SEARCHING AND REVIEWING THE LITERATURE

LEARNING OUTCOMES

On completion of this chapter the reader should be able to:

- appreciate the need to develop literature-searching skills
- define the term 'literature search'
- define the term 'literature review'
- identify sources of research and other forms of evidence
- identify the steps in undertaking a literature search
- understand the need to accurately record and store references.

KEY CONCEPTS

- literature search
- search strategy
- primary source
- literature review
- abstract

- secondary source
- internet
- electronic database
- grey literature

INTRODUCTION

Finding and retrieving literature is an essential skill for all health and social care practitioners. As highlighted previously, it is essential that these professional groups become 'research literate' and this includes having the ability to search for, retrieve, and critically appraise all types of literature in their search for the best evidence. This chapter considers how to find and retrieve literature. This is commonly known as **literature searching**. The chapter will also consider literature reviewing in general terms, and Chapter 11 will consider the **critical appraisal** of different types of literature in some depth.

It is fairly obvious that researchers need to know their subject before embarking on a new piece of research. As Chapter 3 highlighted, in the early stages of the research process it is usual for a researcher to undertake a literature search at the commencement of a study (although with some research designs this does not come at the start). It is also important for the researcher to keep updating the search throughout the life of the study. The reasons for a researcher to undertake a literature search are multiple (see Table 5.1). They include developing a research proposal by getting ideas about methodology, checking that the work has not been undertaken before and extending the researcher's own knowledge about the subject.

Table 5.1   *Reasons for a researcher to undertake a literature search*

- To see if the research question has already been answered.
- To become familiar and knowledgeable about other studies and relevant reports in a particular subject area.
- To gather ideas about appropriate research methodology for their own study, e.g., sample, methods, analysis.
- To see if there are similar studies which could be replicated or refined.
- To enable the researcher to become more focused.
- To assist the researcher in refining the research problem, subject or topic of interest into a clear and specific research question, aim or hypothesis.

The majority of health and social care practitioners are not going to be undertaking research themselves; however, they need to be able to undertake a literature search for a number of reasons (see Table 5.2). Any student embarking on a course today will need to quickly develop highly efficient and effective literature-searching skills. From pre-qualifying through to postgraduate and post-registration courses these skills will be in demand. Being able to search the literature effectively is also essential for **evidence-based practice**. Chapter 2 identified ways in which we 'know' things, and pointed out that these are not always accurate or satisfactory. Finding literature to support or refute what we think we know is one way of developing our knowledge of a subject.

Table 5.2   *Reasons for a practitioner to undertake a literature search*

- To become familiar and knowledgeable about a particular subject.
- To keep abreast of new research and development in a particular subject area.
- As part of an academic assessment, coursework or project work.
- As necessary background work prior to setting standards and developing policy.
- As an important stage in any piece of research.
- As an essential tool for developing professional knowledge and evidence-based practice.

THE LITERATURE SEARCH

A literature search is a process by which a person looks for literature on a specific subject or topic. It needs to be undertaken in a systematic way, and requires time, determination and perseverance. There are a bewildering number of resources available that are constantly being developed, which makes it sometimes difficult to keep up. This chapter can only give a flavour of what is available today. With the 'explosion' of information to support evidence-based practice now available through new technology, both the health and social services are attempting to make access to this information as easy as possible through a single point of access. 'Health Information Resources' and 'Social Care Online' enable free access to information and research to both practitioners and the public.

A number of steps can be followed, and it may be helpful for the 'novice' at literature searching to work through these (see Table 5.3).

People today have access to the internet either at home, through their place of work, in internet cafés and increasingly through mobile technologies, and this will make searching easier,

Table 5.3   *Steps in undertaking a literature search*

- Ensure you have access to online searching, such as databases and the internet.
- Locate suitable libraries that might support your search.
- Become familiar with the variety of sources of literature.
- Become familiar with the range of 'searching facilities' available to you, e.g., electronic resources, indexes, abstracts, websites and current awareness publications.
- Identify key words and develop a search strategy to help you methodically and thoroughly search through abstracts and indexes using the internet.
- Obtain the reports and articles that you want to critically appraise.
- Record the full details and reference of the article or report, including the source.

although libraries will always be necessary for retrieving some literature. One really useful thing to do in the early stages is to use the online introductory guides, workbooks and teaching sessions provided in most university libraries to enable you to get to grips quickly with the range of resources available. Libraries have changed over the past decade and librarians now teach the skills of information retrieval so that health and social care professionals can find information for themselves. Getting to know the librarians and support staff at the beginning of a literature search can also be very fruitful when things get hectic later on in the searching process.

Libraries situated in colleges and universities where there is a department related to one's professional group are likely to have the most useful resources. This will include electronic catalogues, e-books, databases and indexes, as well as access to the internet. There may also be libraries provided by local health and social services, and other local libraries that may be useful. Students will have direct access to their university library and probably limited access to local health and social service libraries. Qualified staff are likely to have limited access to university libraries, which often have arrangements with local organisations in the health and social services. If a library provides a service in subjects such as psychology, biology, sociology, health or social policy, there will be an even wider choice. Professional organisations, such as in nursing, social work and physiotherapy, may also provide services for supporting literature searching, for example, specific databases or electronic books (e-books).

SEARCHING THE LITERATURE

When the researcher has identified the resources available, the next stage is to become familiar with the variety of sources of literature (see Appendix 1). These can be loosely categorised into electronic sources, such as online databases, library catalogues, internet resources such as discussion groups and gateways to sites, e-books, conference papers; and printed sources, such as card catalogues, indexes and **abstracts** in book format. Electronic searching facilities are more accessible and will be more up to date than printed sources and, once the skills have been mastered, are much quicker for searching as they have such comprehensive indexes.

Having become familiar with the range of resources available to search for literature, the researcher must now search through some of the most appropriate sources in a systematic and methodical manner using key words or terms. It is crucial to be clear about the question to which one is seeking an answer, as a vague search for references to heart attack or child abuse will reveal thousands of potential references, most of which will not be relevant. The success of the search can be dependent on choosing the appropriate words and terms and developing a '**search strategy**' (see, for example, Hek et al., 2000). If looking for evidence about 'what works?', a clear question with a number of components might include: type of patient or client; the problem or condition; the intervention or care; and an outcome. For example:

> Does a home-based teaching programme for parents of young children with hyperactivity disorder improve parents' self-esteem and feelings of self-worth?
>
> How soon can patients who have swallowing difficulty following a stroke be safely fed orally?

Each of the components in the questions can be broken down into single words or terms that can then be combined in the search in order to produce only the most 'matched' references. Databases have thesaurus and subject headings to help identify different words to use; so, for instance, a search for a question about cancer might need to include words such as neoplasm and tumour and if it is an American database, alternative spellings might need to be used, for example, tumor. It is beyond this introductory text to go into depth about searching for literature and evidence; suffice to say that these skills are best learnt under the guidance of a librarian who will have extensive knowledge about the latest techniques and sources. Further information can be found in Moule and Goodman (2014).

Other techniques that can be used for literature searching that are less effective, and if used should be in tandem with the main literature search, include: trawling through five years of a specialised journal, for example, *Nursing in Critical Care, British Journal of Occupational Therapy, Journal of Wound Care Journal of Biomechanics, Pain, The British Journal of Social Work;* **snowballing**, which means finding a few key articles, particularly **literature reviews**, then chasing up relevant references from those articles to find others and so on until saturation; general searching on the internet and following up leads; and undertaking a broad search with vague terms, for example, child abuse, and then refining as you go along, rather than being specific right from the start.

SOURCES OF LITERATURE

Primary and secondary sources of information exist. Primary sources are usually published by the researchers who conducted the research, whereas secondary sources make reference to the original, primary source. 'Systematic reviews' are secondary sources. They are systematic collections of available literature on a topic, which have been critically appraised and reviewed and then published. They answer a specific question by summarising the available evidence and are an invaluable source, usually published by a team of systematic reviewers. Probably the most important sources of research literature are the academic and professional journals. Some journals contain original research articles as primary sources, some contain summaries or systematic reviews of research, and many journals publish a mixture including case studies, discussion papers and news items. With the rise of evidence-based practice, there are now some really important journals that specialise in providing a review of research in a specific area, and often provide a commentary about the relevance for practice. They include: *International Journal of Evidence-based Health Care, Evidence-based Mental Health,* and *Evidence-based Medicine.*

Books and e-books will have limited use if the reader is looking for the very latest research. They are very useful for their coverage of a subject in some depth, including research methodology; however, it usually takes a while to get a book published, so it may be a little out of date before it reaches the bookshelves. This may not be important for some readers and for some subjects, but from a research and 'finding the latest evidence' point of view, usually the most recent work is necessary. Some edited books contain recent research on a particular topic, and these can be fairly up-to-date resources.

'Grey literature' includes reports, leaflets, bulletins, circulars and documents that may not be published in the conventional way and therefore will not necessarily show up on electronic literature searches. A wide range of organisations may publish grey literature, including: universities, voluntary organisations, independent research institutions, government departments, funders of research and professional organisations. Some reports might provide a really in-depth account of primary research, or an overview of research findings on a particular topic. Other types of literature might be policy statements, work-in-progress, theses, strategy documents, resource packs, all of which can be rich sources of information to supplement the main literature search.

DEALING WITH THE LITERATURE

In most libraries you can save your search results electronically as a PDF or Word document, and then email them to yourself, or print out the search results. This information will be needed when you write up or refer to the findings of your literature search. Details should include: full name of author(s); date of publication; article title/chapter title/book title/journal title; volume/issue; page numbers; and possibly the Digital Objective Identifier (DoI) number. For books you also need the place of publication, the name of the publisher, edition number and names of editor(s) and possibly the International Standard Book Number (ISBN). This will save a lot of wasted time later when you are trying to find the full details of the reference, that would be required if intending to publish the work. You need to identify those materials that are relevant to you by reviewing the abstracts of articles before either saving or printing them. You will also need to review other potential sources such as books before borrowing. You may need to photocopy any materials not available online, closely observing the copyright regulations. If the item is not available either electronically or in the library, it may be possible to order printed copies from, for example, the British Library. For further help with this see Moule and Goodman (2014).

STORING REFERENCES

It is very useful, and often necessary, to develop a system for storing the references that you obtain. Though a system for computer storage of documents or card filing systems can be created, a number of specific computer programs for storing references can be purchased or may be available through education or work-based libraries. These include Reference Manager, EndNote and ProCite, and they can be extremely useful as they allow you to use the stored references in different ways. For example, you can print out a list of your selected references in a variety of different styles such as the Harvard or Vancouver system. Another way of storing references on a computer is to use a database program. In your storage system you might also like to make notes on each item.

LITERATURE REVIEW

A literature review is a written piece of work that examines and summarises a particular subject in some detail. It may be a large article or paper published as a 'literature review', or a shorter piece that is found at the beginning of a research article. A literature review may perform a number of functions. One function as a result of undertaking a literature search may be to summarise what is written about a particular subject or topic. This might be an uncritical summary that just describes what is written on a particular subject, or more importantly a systematic review which uses explicit, systematic and clearly identified methods to try to reach an unbiased conclusion. The techniques used in a systematic review include critical appraisal of each article or paper (see Chapter 11) and following strict criteria as part of the search strategy.

In order to undertake a critical literature review, the reviewer needs skills to complete a comprehensive literature search (see above) as well as the skills of appraisal. Therefore, knowledge of research methods is essential as well as knowledge of the subject. Most academic assignments expect some critical appraisal of evidence, and for health and social care practitioners, a literature review may underpin the setting of standards or developing guidelines for good practice or for auditing purposes. For the researcher, a critical literature review is essential for informing the research approach and methods of investigating the **research question**. Reviewing the literature is an essential stage in any research process and Moule and Goodman (2014) provide a very readable guide to the process of doing a literature review.

KEY POINTS

- All health and social care practitioners need to develop literature-searching skills.
- Searching for literature is a planned and methodical process with a number of key stages.
- There are numerous sources of literature, including journals, reports and books, often held electronically.
- Indexes and abstracts can help you locate relevant literature.
- Undertaking a thorough literature search requires time, energy and perseverance.

FURTHER READING

Battany-Saltikov, J. (2012). *How to do a systematic review in nursing: A step-by-step guide.* Milton Keynes: RCN.

Hart, C. (1998). *Doing a literature review.* London: Sage.

Hart, C. (2001). *Doing a literature search: A comprehensive guide for the social sciences.* London: Sage.

Hek, G., Langton, H. and Blunden, G. (2000). Systematically searching and reviewing literature. *Nurse Researcher,* 7 (3), 40–57.

Ridley, D. (2012). *The literature review: A step-by-step guide for students* (2nd edn). London: Sage.

WEBSITES

Health Information Resources: www.nhsghpcat.org
National Library for Health: www.evidence.nhs.uk
Social Care Online: www.scie-socialcareonline.org.uk

6 APPROACHES TO AND DESIGN OF RESEARCH IN HEALTH AND SOCIAL CARE

LEARNING OUTCOMES

On completion of this chapter the reader should be able to:

- identify the difference between qualitative and quantitative approaches to research
- describe different approaches under the umbrella of qualitative and quantitative research
- appreciate how research designs such as action research and feminist research may be used as an agent of change and empowerment
- recognise the role played by systematic literature reviews to underpin professional practice.

KEY CONCEPTS

- qualitative
- survey
- feminist research
- mixed methods
- historical research
- systematic reviews
- evaluation research

- quantitative
- experimental/quasi-experimental
- case studies
- consensus methods
- ex post facto
- action research

INTRODUCTION

The research design is the plan that the researchers will follow in order to answer the research aims, objectives, hypothesis and questions. It can be informed by a literature review, where previous study designs may be employed or adapted. The chosen design will include the research approach, ethical considerations, sampling strategy, methods of data collection and analysis. Different research designs and methods can be used within the research approach adopted, which can be presented as either qualitative or quantitative.

QUALITATIVE RESEARCH

Qualitative research is described as being part of an interpretivist approach that can be viewed as constructivist (Guba and Lincoln, 1982). Interpretivists believe that that through interpreting and drawing meaning from the social world, it can be understood. In its crudest sense, qualitative research is attempting to generate data that comprises words and images. The research aims to explore perceptions and experiences in order to understand and explain behaviour. Themes and concepts are developed from an interpretation of mainly observational and interview data. Observational studies in which behaviours are observed and fully recorded are rarely in numerical form. Similarly, focused interviews, in which the researcher holds a 'conversation' with the subjects, produces data that are often described as 'rich' in detail. The research often describes local situations and experiences and can be open to transferability to other settings. Qualitative researchers aim to describe and interpret individuals and their experiences, rather than aspiring to identify a single truth. For example, the approach acknowledges that administrating an injection may elicit a broad range of responses. Qualitative researchers accept that individuals will react to, and experience the injection in different ways and that one person's response will not be representative of a larger group of people.

Qualitative research might include phenomenology, ethnography or grounded theory. Phenomenology is grounded in philosophy and psychology and aims to explore the lived experience of an individual (Beck, 1994). For example, a nurse researcher may want to explore the experience of a group of service users, and consider their perception of the world as a service user and their experiences of the service currently delivered. Ethnography aims to understand the culture and social norms of a particular group, such as carers, by observing behaviours (Hammersley and Atkinson, 2007). Nurse researchers would employ ethnography to gain understanding of the ways in which a local group behave, exist and operate, to understand their world and how it is perceived

(Polit and Beck, 2014). Grounded theory (Glaser and Strauss, 1967) uses data collected through observations and interviews with individuals in their own environment to develop hypotheses and theories. These can be subjected to further observation to explore and verify relationships and correlations.

Qualitative research may require engagement of the researcher in a particular setting for a prolonged period of time. The researcher can become immersed in the study environment, collecting data through a range of methods such as interviews, observations and analysis of diaries, letters and other documents provided by the participants. These methods provide the researcher with in-depth data about personal feelings, experiences and thinking. The researcher may also become an 'instrument' in the research, through reflecting on their role and influence in the study. Researchers often maintain a diary and record field notes, which can form part of the overall data analysis and be included in the final report.

QUANTITATIVE RESEARCH

Quantitative research is described as being part of a positivist or scientific approach, or latterly, a post-positivist approach. The positivist approach stresses the importance of testing, measuring and achieving scientific truth, which might be seen as a 'universal law'. Positivists believe that the truth can be accessed through controlling variables and testing for cause-and-effect relationships. For example, they would assert that patients experiencing pain after a particular procedure would always have that same degree of pain were the procedure repeated and that all patients would have the same level of pain. However, post-positivists accept that 'universal laws' cannot explain social phenomena and that it is problematic to predict a cause-and-effect relationship that applies to everyone. They look for relationships or correlations between variables being measured, such as the relationship between reported pain and preoperative information giving. Quantitative research originated with the work of Fisher (1971), who developed thinking around a hypothesis (a statement of predicted outcome tested by the researcher), guiding the research design and statistical analysis.

Quantitative research can include experimental and correlation studies. Nurse researchers use experimental research designs to test cause–effect relationships (Burns and Grove, 2007). The experimental design has evolved to include quasi-experimental designs used when cause–effect relationships are tested but conditions are less controlled. This design can appeal to social science and health care research, where elements of an experimental design cannot be achieved. For example, it may not be feasible to randomly allocate the study sample to control and experimental groups. Correlation studies aim to identify the strength of relationship between two variables and can be employed to aid the development of a hypothesis (Burns and Grove, 2007). For example, a correlation study may be used to measure the relationship between the number of cigarettes smoked by women in pregnancy and the birth weight of their babies.

Quantitative research might be thought of as any type of research in which measurement is involved. The term 'quantitative' may refer to both the method of collecting the data and the type of data involved. The criteria revolve around whether or not the data are already in numerical form or can be easily transformed into numbers.

In its basic form this numerical data will include the frequency in which a **phenomenon** occurs. At the more sophisticated end of the scale exact measurements will be recorded under very strict conditions. The importance of recognising the characteristics of these different levels of measurement is emphasised and discussed fully in Chapter 10. The data collection methods most frequently employed in quantitative research include the use of **questionnaires** and structured **interviews**.

In order to produce data collecting tools or instruments, which will accurately measure the phenomena being studied, the researcher will need to have considerable knowledge of the subject/ phenomena under scrutiny. A frequent criticism of **quantitative data collection** is that there is not enough evidence that the data collection tool is actually measuring the phenomena under study. The purpose of such research is often to test a theory through observation or the development of testing, with the ultimate aim of generalising and applying the results to a wide population.

ADDITIONAL CONSIDERATIONS

Classifying research as qualitative and quantitative identifies a research approach and, possibly more relevant, a type of data collection and subsequent analysis. Although usually presented as fairly 'tight' compartments, studies may include different methods of data collection, which encompass both categories. In some cases researchers purposely use more than one approach to investigate a phenomenon. The term '**triangulation**' may be used to describe studies which collect data in different ways (data triangulation) or use different researchers (researcher triangulation). In essence, the use of triangulation adds weight to the findings.

Sometimes research studies are categorised according to their location. The terms 'field' and 'laboratory' studies are sometimes used and both have their advantages and disadvantages. Similarly, case studies may be conducted in a single centre, and phenomena examined from several positions using more than one research approach.

Instead of collecting their own data researchers may use existing facts and figures collected by another agency. National archives may hold data collected by various organisations, such as academic and government departments, to which researchers may have access. This type of research can provide social researchers with an opportunity to study large-scale data sets using limited resources. With most organisations now using computerised information systems, the amount of data potentially available for researchers is increasing all the time. In an effort to utilise the results from many small studies, **meta-analysis** is also recognised as a legitimate way of re-analysing quantitative data to produce more meaningful results.

In designing a study the researcher may have to consider the **concept** of time and location. In this chapter various research designs, such as prospective study (looking ahead), **retrospective study** (looking backwards), *ex post facto* (after an event) and historical designs, will be discussed. As part of the prospective studies, cross-sectional and **longitudinal research** will also be examined.

The selection of a research design will also be influenced by a number of practical issues. The researcher will need to consider the resources available, such as time, funding and researcher skills or expertise. A restricted budget may impact on, for example, the design and the data collection methods used.

QUALITATIVE DESIGNS

Qualitative research usually starts with a set of observations of a situation. From this early stage the researcher would plan to document the information very carefully. This approach in research encapsulates the philosophy that people are fundamentally different from things, and should be valued as individuals. As patterns of behaviour or interactions develop the researcher seeks to make sense of them from the individual's perspective.

When undertaking qualitative research there are several points that the researcher must be clear about regarding the approach to data collection. Initially, whatever data collection methods are used, great effort must be made by the researcher not to influence the collection of data. This research approach demands that the picture painted is as close to the real situation as possible and that no attempt is made at interpretation. In the observational account, the physical environment is often described, as well as the speech and actions of individuals, so that a complete picture is painted.

In undertaking qualitative research a researcher may have certain beliefs about the individual in society. Burns and Grove (2013) suggest that there is a need for 'methodological congruence', or 'fit', between the research design and the researcher's philosophical orientation.

ETHNOGRAPHY

This approach has its roots in social anthropology, when researchers lived among the group of individuals being studied. The term 'going native' was coined from these early studies and the work of ethnographers such as Mead who, in the 1930s, lived among tribes in Papua New Guinea (Haralambos and Holborn, 2008). In more modern times 'going native' might refer to joining groups that are being studied, such as football supporters or a group of homeless individuals. Whatever group is being studied, the crucial point is that of becoming an 'insider', and experiencing the group or organisation 'as one of them', and not as an 'outsider' looking in.

In order to be able to study a group in such depth, the researcher has to enter the study without preconceptions about the group or the questions to be asked. Through **observations** and in-depth questioning, the researcher looks for connections, patterns and themes that have meaning for the people within that culture. These themes might include shared belief systems, language, or role behaviours.

PRACTICE EXAMPLE

Ethnographic studies have been used to examine relationships and roles within health and social care, with researchers taking 'insider' researcher roles. One example is a study completed by Thomson (2011), which explored the everyday lives of health professionals. This

(Continued)

(Continued)

study included many of the aspects of ethnographic design highlighted above, such as being an 'insider' with an understanding and familiarity of the setting that allowed a shared understanding of context, language and roles, and data collection through observation. Thomson was a senior lecturer with experience of physiotherapy practice at the time of the study. Having knowledge of physiotherapy helped Thomson to understand the organisational and policy contexts that the health care professionals were working in. Thomson collected data using observations and interviews, but also used a reflexive approach, recording field notes and using these to reflect on her own position within the research, as well as to inform the ongoing data collection. Thomson notes the effectiveness of the approach employed over a prolonged period of time, which allowed an in-depth exploration of the practice of health care professionals.

PHENOMENOLOGY

Phenomenology has its roots in European philosophy, and is based on knowledge gained from the experiences of the individual and the individual's view of the world. In this approach the research question is explained through 'lived experiences' as described by those being studied. There is a basic belief by the researcher that individuals have attitudes, values and knowledge with which they make sense of their world and which guide their actions. Burns and Grove (2013) argue that phenomenologists view the individual as integral with their environment and that every experience is unique. Therefore the role of phenomenology is to describe the experience being studied rather than attempt to define or explain it. In general the researcher strives to capture the richness of the experience while maintaining a strong orientation to the fundamental research question (van Manen, 1990).

PRACTICE EXAMPLE

Langfield and James (2009) used a qualitative phenomenological approach to explore the ownership of fish as pets. The approach was chosen because the study aimed to explore the meaning of how humans experience the phenomenon of owning a fish as a pet and to do this through gathering the descriptions of experiences of ownership as lived by the individuals. The study received ethical approval and used data collection methods consistent with the phenomenological approach. Data was collected through in-depth, semi-structured interviews. The data allowed the researcher to gain an in-depth understanding of the meaning of fish ownership from the perspective of the fish owner. The sample was selected to reflect inclusion criteria. These were: lived locally, aged over 18, and currently owning and caring for one or more pet fish in a tank/aquarium. The sampling strategy used was a snowball technique (see Chapter 8), using initial contacts to identify other participants. In interviewing the nine participants, the researchers used open-ended questions to allow the participants to provide a rich description of their experiences as fish owners. One of the researchers had also owned a fish previously. In presenting the research, the team commented that this enabled the researcher to relate some of the participants' experiences to her own and 'facilitated deeper exploration of the issues raised' (Langfield and James, 2009: 352). The interview data was transcribed to give a verbatim (word-for-word) account of the conversation. These were analysed by each researcher independently coding the data to develop themes through a constant comparative method (see Chapter 10). The participants undertook 'member checking' by discussing the themes that the researchers identified from the data. This helped to ensure the researchers were presented with the 'lived experiences' of the participants and that their analysis reflected the participants' experiences of fish ownership.

GROUNDED THEORY

Grounded theory as an approach to research was initially developed by Glaser and Strauss (1967) and has been further developed by Strauss and Corbin (1998). Glaser and Strauss (1967) generated a systematic procedure for developing a theory about a phenomenon from the collected data. As the researcher examines the data, which have been collected by observations or interviews, themes and concepts are identified. The researcher then returns frequently to the data, looking for further evidence of the themes and revising the research question as issues arise from the data.

To use grounded theory, the researcher needs to have knowledge of the literature and people's experience of the situation being examined. The literature is used to provide the researcher with prompts and guidance to the concepts related to the area under investigation. In many ways, grounded theory is perceived as the far end of the inductive continuum as theories are actually produced. In phenomenology and **ethnography** the themes and categories describing behaviours in their social context are often the end point of the study.

PRACTICE EXAMPLE

Kelly and Nisker (2010) used a grounded theory approach to develop a theoretical model of medical students' responses to patient death. The study included final year medical students, collecting data through individual interviews, focus groups and via email. The recorded data was transcribed and verbatim transcripts and email text were analysed. The process of analysis included three different stages of coding that are often used in grounded theory analysis: open, axial and selective coding (see Strauss and Corbin, 1998). The initial open coding identified 28 categories, which were then explored to identify relationships across the data, presented as overarching themes. A final stage of analysis looked at the way in which the overarching themes interacted. There were three overlying themes: (1) young, (2) old and (3) unexpected deaths. The seven themes identified at axial coding were (1) preparation, (2) the death event, (3) feelings, (4) the role of the clinical clerk, (5) differential factors between deaths, (6) closure and (7) relationships. The researchers used these themes to develop a model of students' experiences of death identified at selective coding level that included: preparation, the event itself, the crisis, the resolution, and the lessons learnt.

EVALUATION RESEARCH

Evaluation research focuses on collecting data to ascertain the effects of some form of planned change or intervention, such as policy, practice or service (Lincoln and Guba, 1986). It is growing increasingly important in health care as there is pressure to demonstrate the effectiveness of interventions and procedures to ensure the best quality of care is provided and that resources are used in the most effective and efficient way (Moule and Goodman, 2014).

Evaluation research aims to find out whether a particular policy or intervention is working and is often linked to audit in health services. There is, however, an important difference between audit and evaluation research. Audit is used to record the extent of change, often measuring against pre-set standards, whereas evaluation seeks to explore what has changed and why (Moule and Goodman, 2014).

Evaluation research might be applied to look at the effects of a new policy initiative in the NHS, such as the effect of new roles in radiotherapy (for example, the sonographer), or the impact of assistant practitioner roles in the allied health professions. In researching the effectiveness of new roles, the outcomes of the research would aim to help policy-makers in the NHS decide whether these new roles should be extended, changed or completely replaced. The research focus is therefore to evaluate the effects of change in practice brought about by new policy or initiatives, rather than to generate new knowledge. The research designs employed by researchers can include qualitative and quantitative methods.

QUANTITATIVE DESIGNS

In quantitative research a prediction is made of the presence, or not, of a difference or a relationship between two or more factors (usually referred to as **variables**). The prediction is made through a **hypothesis** or measurable statement developed from a theory. This prediction will then be tested. The results of the research will either support the prediction or not, thereby confirming the theory or not.

In essence, quantitative research depends on several considerations to withstand scrutiny. The first requirement is that there must be an existing theory on which to base the hypothesis and give the study a focus. Following that, a previously tested data-collecting tool will be needed to collect information from a **representative sample** of the research population. The analysis of the results will demand rigorous statistical testing in which the possibility of these results occurring by chance will be demonstrated and discussed. Quantitative research tends to be tightly managed and highly structured, to allow the movement of the findings from the specific sample to a more general research population. This movement is sometimes referred to as the **generalisability** of the results.

SURVEYS

Surveys are widely used to collect information from a large number of people. They are primarily designed to study the relationship and incidence of variables in a population, such as attitudes and values and demographic details: for example, age and type of living accommodation. Questionnaires are frequently used to collect this information, with the respondent completing a self-administered form and returning it to the researcher. A telephone may also be used, and the respondents' replies noted immediately. Telephone surveys allow the researcher to 'interview' a large sample of individuals from a wide geographical area. However, there can be drawbacks. The researcher has to acknowledge that telephone calls need to be pre-arranged to be most effective, as otherwise a number of people will just put the phone down, and those who have hearing difficulties may need to be excluded from the sample (as do those without a telephone). Online surveys or surveys sent to mobile devices are becoming increasingly popular. They are quick to administer and can access participants world-wide in a short time frame. There are some disadvantages, however, as email address accuracy must be ensured. Emails can be easily deleted, affecting response rates. Furthermore, in surveys, face-to-face interviews can be used, where the researcher tends to obtain more information and a high rate of returns as few people refuse to be interviewed. However, it is a time-consuming procedure, and the sample would be much smaller than that used with a questionnaire.

There are two main types of survey: descriptive and correlational. In descriptive surveys, data are collected from a sample of individuals and the results describe the situation as the researchers find it. For example, in a survey of social work students who qualified in 2010 the researcher might describe the number who now work in social services, those who work in the independent sector and those who do not practice. There is no further analysis beyond the description. Descriptive surveys can be cross-sectional if data are collected from one sample at one point in time, or longitudinal if conducted at more than one time. A correlational survey goes further. In this type of survey the results include a description of the findings. The researcher then seeks to find relationships between the characteristics (variables) in which they are interested, such as whether social workers have taken up posts with children and young people.

PRACTICE EXAMPLE

The use of online data collection techniques can be attractive to researchers as they reach a geographically diverse group within a short time frame. Responses can also be collated electronically, which saves resources. The method has therefore been used by a number of researchers, including Bruns et al. (2012). They wanted to access physicians at three different sites across Brazil. A total of 41,847 physicians were invited to take part in the survey by email. The survey asked 21 questions. These related to what measurements were being undertaken of the fetal heart, as part of routine scanning in pregnancy. The final analysis included a sample of 467. The use of the online survey therefore achieved access to a wide sample through email, and attracted responses from across Brazil. The researchers had considered ethical issues and provided opportunities for online informed consent. Whilst the final sample size was lower than might have been expected, the response rate provided sufficient data for analysis.

EXPERIMENTAL/QUASI-EXPERIMENTAL DESIGNS IN RESEARCH

The ability of the researcher to control or manipulate elements of the study renders experimental research different from other approaches (Moule and Goodman, 2014). In experimental research the researcher is interested in the effect of different treatments on two or more groups, which have been matched. Usually this means manipulating the **independent variable** (or cause) and examining and measuring the **dependent variable** (or effect).

In true experimental research the investigator is an active agent who has responsibility in three specific areas:

1. Randomisation – subjects are assigned to the experimental or **control group** in a randomised manner. Everyone in the study must have an equal chance of being included in any group.
2. Control – there must be a control group who receive the traditional or usual care/treatment.
3. Manipulation – the researcher must have an **experimental group** receiving different care/treatment.

When these three conditions are stringently applied, the results of true **experiments** in examining a causal relationship are most powerful.

Although the results of experiments are powerful there are many problems in using them. The ethical considerations associated with using human beings in experiments limits their use. Moule and Goodman (2014) also suggest that a problem with using experiments can be that of the **'hawthorne effect'**, in which people alter their behaviour when they know they are part of a study.

When this happens the results of the experiment might be affected.

Because of these problems in conducting experiments the notion of **quasi-experiments** has been developed. There is still the manipulation of the independent variable, but there may be limited randomisation, or use of a control group. The results of quasi-experiments are therefore considerably weaker than those of true experiments. The term 'quasi-experiments' is also used to describe experimental studies which lack one or more of the conditions noted above.

In the most controlled settings a laboratory may be used. It may not look like a traditional laboratory as, in some studies, buildings have been made to look like prisons or hospital wards in order to set up an experiment.

An alternative to a laboratory experiment is to use a field approach. In this type of experiment the research is conducted wherever the subjects are likely to be found, such as in a clinic, a hospital ward or in the street. Often field experiments are quasi-experiments, as it is difficult to control all variables. Experiments which take place in practice settings involving patients/clients are commonly called randomised control trials (RCTs). The trial can be referred to as a 'single blind trial' when the researchers are unaware of which group the patient is in, but the patient and their carers know their group. In trials where no one involved with the experiment knows which group the participants are in (for example, drug trials where placebos are used) the term 'double blind' is used.

PRACTICE EXAMPLE

Research undertaken by Silva et al. (2010) used a randomised control trial design. The researchers were keen to see whether behaviour change interventions were effective in promoting physical exercise and weight control in women. They started by accessing a total sample of 239 women who had to meet a series of inclusion criteria. They had, for example, to be aged between 25 and 50 years, not be pregnant, have a body mass index of between 25 and 40 kg/m² and be free from major illnesses. This meant that the researchers limited some of the factors that might have affected the results, such as very big differences in weight. The 239 women were then randomised into one of two groups, meaning that the researchers didn't choose which women went into which group: the women could have been placed in either. The groups were an experimental group, who received the intervention based on self-determination theory that promoted autonomous forms of exercise and intrinsic motivation, and the control group, who were offered general health improvement programmes. The researchers therefore used an accepted RCT design. They had a control group who received a more standard treatment and they manipulated the treatment of the experimental group, who received the self-determination theory-based programme. Measurements of weight and exercise taken at various points over a 12-month period were compared using statistical tests to look for a difference between the groups. The researchers found that the women in the experimental group showed increased weight loss and higher levels of physical activities when compared to the control group. This suggested that the self-determination theory-based programme could be used to support weight loss and promote physical activity.

EX POST FACTO RESEARCH DESIGNS

Ex post facto literally means 'after the fact'. In these studies there is an investigation about a relationship between two or more variables, but after the events have been allowed to happen. The two most common forms of *ex post facto* research designs are retrospective and prospective studies. In retrospective studies the researcher wants to study an effect, and will search for some causative factor of that effect. Prospective studies are conducted in the light of presumed causes. Researchers will follow their subjects forward in time and look for an effect which is due to the presumed cause. Prospective studies are usually expensive and time consuming because of the need to follow up subjects but they do allow the researcher a greater degree of control.

FEMINIST RESEARCH

From its beginnings as research conducted by feminists, feminist research has developed into a research methodology in its own right. Feminist research attempts to redress the balance of many years of male dominance in explanations of what happens in our society. It does this by developing a non-threatening, non-hierarchical relationship between the researcher and the subjects, and by making women the focus of the study. Feminism focuses on reclaiming and renaming women's experiences and challenging male dominance in establishing the 'truth' through research (Kitzinger, 2004). There is an argument regarding the position of men conducting feminist research. In principle some believe it possible (Harding, 1987, cited by Webb, 1993); others believe that men, by not undergoing a woman's experience, are unable to conduct the research from a woman's position (Kremer, 1990, cited by Webb, 1993). Feminist research is described as: giving attention to the significance of gender; raising women's issues; rejecting the concept of objectivity; recognising the exploitation of women; and empowering women as a result of research (Cook and Fonow, 1986).

As a methodology, feminist research is not constrained by a particular data-collecting method. However, the very nature of feminist research in which there is involvement of the researcher with the researched, and a sharing of experiences, would imply a need for a more open research approach rather than a closed approach.

ACTION RESEARCH

Action research is an approach that attempts to bring about a change in practice. This occurs through action, and reflection on that action, theory and practice, often in participation with others as part of a process of finding solutions to problems of concern (Reason and Bradbury, 2001). Action research tries to bridge the gap that can open up between theory generation and practice change. Researchers using this approach tend to work in a more participatory way with practitioners to develop answers to problems of day-to-day working in health and social care through a cyclical process that uses research methods to assess the problem, plan and implement change and evaluate the outcome to identify further practice issues. Thus, the initial action research approach has developed and changed to take a more participatory focus and if used in this way can be described as participatory action research.

Holloway and Wheeler (2002) suggest action research has a number of unique properties:

- The researchers collaborate with local participants or are themselves in the research setting as 'insider' researchers.
- There is action in the research.
- The process will include problem identification, research, intervention and a change in practice.
- The research findings are implemented in practice and the effect of this is measured (adapted from Holloway and Wheeler, 2002: 189).

Action research attempts to influence the real world by identifying these changes as they take place rather than generating theories. However, there is an argument that action research should begin by observations, either completed in a prior study, or as a preliminary to the action research in which theories may have been generated.

Hanson and Clarke (2000) recognise that although action research has traditionally been placed within a qualitative classification it actually spans a much wider base. They demonstrate the qualities of action research as a means of evaluating the introduction of new services to enhance the autonomy, independence and quality of life of frail older people in the community.

CASE STUDIES

Case study research is growing in popularity, as it allows researchers to conduct small-scale studies around a specific situation. For example, in a study which investigated the care of patients with dementia in hospital, a specific patient might be the 'case' and the researcher would use qualitative and quantitative approaches to investigate all aspects of care, including the role of each member of the multidisciplinary team, communication systems around the care delivered, or the role of social workers in supporting the family. In another example, a school might be the 'case', and all aspects of the school would be investigated, perhaps examining why one school had a higher truancy rate than another. An in-depth discussion of the use of case studies may be found in Bergen and While (2000) and Gomm et al. (2000).

PRACTICE EXAMPLE

Case studies often form part of a mixed methods approach (see below) in order to gain local insight. One example is research undertaken by Moule et al. (2010). The study was looking at the use of e-learning In higher education institutions providing education to health sciences and practice students. The first phase of the project was a survey completed by local staff. This informed sampling for a second phase that used case studies. In total nine universities were used as cases to explore the development and implementation of

(Continued)

(Continued)

e-learning. The survey provided an overall view of the range of e-technologies used and the frequency of use. It also provided information on proposed developments. However, the case studies allowed more in-depth exploration of a range of issues, such as how development was funded and supported, as well as experiences of staff and students in the use of e-learning. Data was collected from staff through individual interviews and from student focus groups and this enabled a more 'close and personal' view of the case sites.

CONSENSUS METHODS

These methods are used to establish a common agreement between, for example, health care team members, in situations where there is no agreed understanding of a health care issue. The method could be used to generate research questions or in the development of new services. There are three commonly used methods in health; Delphi technique, nominal group technique and consensus technique.

The Delphi technique would involve expert panels whose members are engaged in completing a series of questionnaires in order to achieve an agreement or overall view. An initial open questionnaire is composed that allow the experts to report ideas, views and attitudes. Feedback is collated and used to construct a more focused questionnaire, which includes a number of statements related to key topics. The experts are asked to rank their level of agreement with each statement. The results are summarised and returned to the experts in a further questionnaire used to establish a consensus. The process relies on the development of questions that will help the researchers to address the issue, the selection of appropriate unbiased experts and can suffer from engagement fatigue with increased reluctance to engage as the process continues, resulting in poor response rates.

PRACTICE EXAMPLE

Consensus techniques are often used to secure expert agreement on health care issues where there is no agreed understanding. Shaw et al.

(2014) employed the Delphi technique to bring experts together to consider how best to identify when a child might be moving into the latter stages of end-of-life care. The experts involved represented a range of palliative care professionals working with children. An initial questionnaire was developed following a literature review and focus group discussion. It included 75 symptoms that might alert a professional to a change in the child, indicating they may be moving into the final weeks of end-of-life care. The initial questionnaire was completed by 50 experts and a second questionnaire by 49, showing a high level of expert participation. The signs and symptoms that were identified as most likely to indicate end-of-life had a high degree of consensus and were used to inform practice.

The nominal group technique uses some of the principle and processes of the Dephi technique and combines these with a focus group method (see Chapter 9). Consensus is achieved through face-to-face focus group meetings, where experts rank and refine responses to key issues.

Consensus techniques bring panels of experts together in a meeting to establish a consensus and develop clinical practice guidelines. Prior to the panel meeting evidence is collated, through a systematic review of the literature and possible scoping studies (this may include a review of guidelines or practices used elsewhere). This evidence is made available to the experts and informs the discussions.

HISTORICAL RESEARCH

Historical research has the goal of attaining new knowledge from the systematic collection and critical evaluation of data that relates to past events. Polit and Beck (2014) suggest this research approach can primarily use qualitative data and that it examines causes, effects and trends of past events, considering how they might inform present behaviours and practices. Sources of data include documents, records, eyewitness accounts and oral histories. Kirby (2004) used a historical approach to provide an understanding of the range of views about the current position and future of nursing research. Documentary sources used included government reports and professional journals from the 1950s, 1960s and 1970s; these years are seen as the foundation periods for nursing research.

SYSTEMATIC REVIEWS

Increasingly, systematic reviews of previously published research are being written and used by health and social care workers. A systematic review is regarded as secondary research because it analyses existing research findings rather than collecting new data (Parahoo, 2014). The aim of systematic research is to assess all of the available research on a particular topic. The eight stages of a systematic review are explained in Moule and Goodman (2014) and highlight the importance of working with a clear research question and systematic processes of data collection and review. As an exemplar of this process, the **Cochrane Library** databases can be accessed to inform the reader of the results of a systematic review of randomised controlled trials on various topics. However, there are also many examples of systematic reviews in the health and social care literature which take a much wider remit and consider both qualitative and quantitative studies. Many institutions of higher education use **systematic literature reviews** as a basis for dissertation work. The required skills of **critical appraisal** and research synthesis are considered to be as important as collecting and analysing small data sets. An example of systematic review of the treatment for acute bronchiolitis for paediatric patients between 0 and 24 months old can be found in the work of Perrotta et al. (2005). In this review the researchers included papers from a number of databases. It was highlighted that chest physiotherapy using vibration and percussion techniques did not reduce the length of hospitalised stay or oxygen requirements.

META-ANALYSES

Similar to systematic literature reviews are meta-analyses. However, in this case the actual findings of reviewed quantitative studies are amalgamated and reworked. This process can be helpful when there are many small studies on a topic, which on their own are too small to demonstrate an effect but which can produce substantial results when analysed together. It may be possible to draw conclusions when looking at the data from a number of studies, when it would not have been possible from each individual study. They can also aid in gaining a consensus and agreement on best practice when there are inconsistencies in the results of published studies. This approach was used by Kent et al. (2005), who compared the quantitative outcomes of ten randomised controlled trials to explore the effects of mobilisation and manipulation in the treatment of non-specific low back pain. They looked at research where the clinician was either able or unable to select a specific treatment. The findings of the meta-analysis suggested that the ability to tailor manual therapy treatment to the individual was not likely to have a positive impact on patient outcomes. Polit and Beck (2014) provide further explanations of this research approach.

MIXED METHODS

Mixed methods designs combine research methods to address research questions. Triangulating the methods of data collection allows the researcher to compare findings collected in different ways. For example, the results of individual interviews with staff about a particular practice might be compared with the findings of observations on that practice and with written records. To triangulate the data, three or more methods of collecting information are used in the same study (see Chapter 9).

Using different data collection methods to address research questions allows the researcher to gain different perspectives from the data and gives a fuller view and broader research understanding. It is preferable that the methods used are drawn from both qualitative and quantitative traditions. Given the scope of **mixed methods** research its use is increasing in health and social care studies.

PRACTICE EXAMPLE

Mixed methods were used in a study by Mirza et al. (2009) to explore the management of intellectual disabilities in communities in Pakistan. The researchers used multiple methods of data collection to try and reduce the limitations of using just one approach. The carers of people with intellectual disabilities were surveyed (n = 100) using qualitative and quantitative tools. In-depth interviews were conducted with carers (n = 16) and with key primary health care workers (n = 10). Finally, focus groups were conducted (n = 7). The researcher team concluded that using multiple methods of data collection was an effective way of

(Continued)

(Continued)

validating the findings. Their conclusions were based on the different sets of data rather than one, reducing the likelihood of the research making false claims based on one method. It should be noted, however, that the project was more resource intensive, and took longer to complete, than a single design approach.

KEY POINTS

- The selection of the overall research approach must be appropriate to the study and can be described as qualitative, quantitative or a triangulation of both.
- Qualitative research is part of an interpretivist position.
- Quantitative research is part of a positivist position.
- Consensus methods are used to establish a common agreement between experts.
- Action research attempts to change practice while the research is ongoing.
- Feminist research has a particular approach, and is not tied to a specific data collecting method.
- Research can employ mixed methods.

FURTHER READING

Bryderup, I. (2008). *Evidence based and knowledge based social work: Research methods and approaches in social work.* Aarhus: Aarhus University Press.

Gilbert, N. (ed.) (2008). *Researching social life* (3rd edn). London: Sage.

Gomm, R., Hammersley, M. and Foster, P. (eds) (2000). *Case study method.* London: Sage.

Hicks, C. (2009). *Research methods for clinical therapists: Applied project design and analysis* (5th edn). London: Churchill Livingstone.

Hughes, C. (2002). *Key concepts in feminist theory and research.* London: Sage.

McNiff, J. (2010). *You and your action research project* (3rd edn). London: Routledge.

Polit, D. and Beck, C. (2014). *Essentials of nursing research: Appraising evidence for nursing practice* (8th edn). Philadelphia, PA: Lippincott Williams and Wilkins.

Wilkinson, G. (2005). Illustrating triangulation in mixed-methods research. *Nurse Researcher,* 12 (4), 7–18.

WEBSITE

Journal of Mixed Methods Research: http://mmr.sagepub.com

7 RESEARCH PROBLEMS, AIMS, QUESTIONS AND HYPOTHESES

LEARNING OUTCOMES

On completion of this chapter the reader should be able to:

- appreciate the nature of research problems
- understand the formation of research questions
- recognise the difference between research questions and hypotheses
- identify independent and dependent variables.

KEY CONCEPTS

- dependent variable
- null hypotheses
- hypothesis

- research problem
- independent variable
- research question

INTRODUCTION

The health and social care professions demand that practice should influence the identification of problems and questions that are researchable. These 'problems' may have their foundation in the experience and professional practice of individuals, or they may emerge from an existing theory. Researchable problems could also come from the results of previous published research that has identified some new problems or areas that need further research.

In many instances, a problem in practice is identified locally by a health and social care practitioner who feels that something is 'not quite right'. However, they may not feel in any position to do something about the problem. Occasionally this will lead directly to a research project being undertaken. More commonly, health and social care practitioners will be required to review all previously published research and critically appraise it. This will enable the practitioner to look at the problem and consider ways to overcome it.

Other chapters have considered the skills needed by health and social care practitioners to retrieve and critically appraise research findings and literature, and Chapter 3 deliberates upon the research process. This chapter examines research questions, aims and hypotheses, and takes up the position that nursing research questions often arise from problems in practice.

RESEARCH PROBLEMS

Health and social care practitioners need to understand and identify research problems, which can then form the basis of a researchable question. They may not necessarily be involved in undertaking the research. However, they have an important role in identifying researchable questions and setting the agenda for research in practice.

Research problems may also be generated by large organisations that, in turn, identify priorities for research. The National Institute for Health and Care Excellence (NICE), for example, produces clinical guidelines and having already reviewed all the available evidence will then say where there is a gap in the evidence and a need for further research in specific areas. For some organisations, such as the Department of Health, research priorities will be identified and funding awarded for appropriate studies that address the problems.

At an early stage in the research process, a researcher needs to refine the problem into a clear researchable question or questions. The way in which a **research question** is interpreted, however, is dependent on the beliefs, values, experience and approach of the researcher. When reading research, all health and social care practitioners should be aware of the researcher's influence in the way that research questions have been developed from the research problem.

As identified in Chapter 6, there are two broad approaches in research: quantitative research and qualitative research. Quantitative research will use methods of data collection and analysis to test a theory. On the basis of a theory, and prior to data collection, researchers will make predictions about what will happen in specific situations. Qualitative research, however, will use methods of data collection and analysis with the aim of examining the data for patterns and relationships. The purpose is to understand and describe what is going on, with a view to generating a theory. Predictions may be generated from the data and tested and re-tested during the course of the research. However, research using this approach will not usually begin with a prediction of what will be found.

RESEARCH AIMS AND OBJECTIVES

Many researchers identify aims and objectives at the beginning of their study. These will guide the researcher and give some indication of what the researcher is trying to achieve. Aims and objectives are not particularly specific; indeed, they may be intentionally vague. They may identify the purpose of the research, and they may suggest goals or outcomes in quite general terms. However, they do not give a clear indication of what questions are being asked, and they do not make any prediction of what they are expecting to find. Both qualitative and quantitative studies may incorporate research aims and objectives.

RESEARCH QUESTIONS

In order to be able to manage a research project the details of the study need to be made much more explicit, and this is often made clear through the research question(s). Some studies will have more than one research question, or there may be a principal question, followed by a few questions that are more specific. If there is more than one question, they must be clearly related. Most research will have research question(s) posed at the outset of the study, and qualitative studies will continue to be guided by the questions. Exploratory studies, in particular, will identify research questions, occasionally with a view to generating and testing a theory from the descriptive findings of the study.

Clearly articulating and defining the research question is often identified as one of the most difficult stages in the research process (Moule and Goodman, 2014). A good research question needs to be clear and focus on what exactly needs to be known.

Any **variables** stated in the question must be capable of observation and measurement. A research question can either be a statement in question form, or a statement of purpose: 'What is the relationship between the provision of post-registration education and the retention of staff?' or 'The purpose of this study is to investigate the relationship between the provision of post-registration education and the retention of staff.' Further examples of research questions are provided in Table 7.1. The following journals have examples of research aims, questions and hypotheses: *British Medical Journal, International Journal of Nursing Studies, Journal of Advanced Nursing,* and *Journal of Radiotherapy Practice and Physiotherapy.*

Table 7.1   *Examples of research questions*

- Do youth programmes ease the burden on police services of attending youth-related disturbances in the community?
- What are the nursing practice challenges for army nurses in military operations?
- How can the barriers to involving people with dementia in research be addressed?
- Is e-learning as effective in developing student knowledge in resuscitation as classroom-based teaching?
- What are midwives' perceived views on the rate of domestic violence in the UK?

When reading research reports, health and social care practitioners need to be able to identify the source of the research question(s), and how it has been developed from the problem. In some reports, only the problem is identified through a problem statement. If this is the case, the problem needs to clearly identify and define the research variables and the nature of the population being studied. In other types of research, neither the problem nor the research question will be identified. However, there should be a specific purpose to the study which identifies why the study is being conducted.

DEVELOPING RESEARCH AIMS AND QUESTIONS

All researchers will need to formulate research questions, and often aims and hypotheses at the start of a study, as may health care students undertaking their own **literature reviews** or research projects as part of professional courses and study. It is therefore important to follow a framework to support question formulation. This is explained more fully in Moule and Goodman (2014: 91) and put more succinctly here it includes the following:

1. Identify the research problem from practice or other sources.
2. Use the literature search and review (see Chapter 5) to confirm a focused problem that can be researched.
3. Identify what the research aims are – what you aim to do in the research – using words such as: describe, explore, develop, understand, reflect, explain, measure, compare.
4. Develop the root of the question(s): who, what, why, where, when, how, do, is, are?
5. Write short, concise research question(s).
6. Test these out with colleagues, other researchers, fellow students or research facilitators.
7. Refine the question(s).

For additional guidance on how to start a project and the process of turning an idea into a research question see the RDInfo website (http://rdinfo.leeds.ac.uk/Newsletter/Handout.pdf).

As part of the process of developing the research question the researcher should consider a number of factors. For example, is it possible to answer the question(s), are the time and resources available, is there the supervision and support needed for the project, and are there ethical issues in pursuing the answer to the question? The feasibility of the study may also be affected by other factors such as access to the sample group and resources.

PRACTICE EXAMPLE

To demonstrate the development of a research question, we can look at the work of Moule et al. (2010), and the processes taken that relate to the above framework for developing research questions.

1. The research problem was identified by the funding body and formed the basis of a research tendering process. The problem was a lack of knowledge about how e-learning was being developed and used by universities delivering health sciences and practice education.

(Continued)

(Continued)

2. A literature search was undertaken by the research team that confirmed and refined the problem and informed the development of the research question that needed to be answered in the study.
3. The study aimed to scope e-learning and teaching implementation in health sciences and practice disciplines throughout universities in the UK and explore those issues influencing implementation and use.
4. There was the need for more than one question to address the aim. The possible question roots were 'How', 'What'.
5. Possible research questions:

   • 'How are higher education institutions developing and using e-learning to support the educational preparation of health sciences and practice students?'
   • 'What factors affect the development and use of e-learning technologies by higher education institutions?'

6. These questions were agreed by the funding body and research team.

RESEARCH HYPOTHESES

In some approaches to research, a **hypothesis** is devised before the study begins and this will guide the whole study. The hypothesis goes further than a research question and is directly related to the research problem. It is used primarily, although not exclusively, in quantitative studies. The hypothesis is a statement about the relationship between two or more variables and predicts an expected outcome. Variables are any characteristics about a person that can vary: age, sex, height, eye colour, etc. In some studies, the variables need to be clearly defined because they are not always obvious. The hypothesis will also determine who and what is to be studied, and the way that the findings are interpreted.

Unlike a research question, a hypothesis will predict what will happen in a particular study and it can be a very powerful and persuasive tool.

At the end of a study, a research question never permits the investigator to say more than: 'This is how the world looked when I observed it.' In contrast, hypotheses permit the investigator to say: 'Based on my particular explanation about how the world works, this is what I expected to observe, and behold – that is exactly how it looked! For that reason my explanation of how the world works must be given credibility.' When a hypothesis is confirmed, the investigator is empowered to make arguments about knowledge that go far beyond what is available when a question has been asked and answered.

A hypothesis can also be stated as a **'null' hypothesis**. The null hypothesis states that there is no relationship between the variables. The null hypothesis is the preferred approach in some quantitative studies and is associated with tests of **statistical significance**. Hypotheses and null hypotheses are never 'proved' or 'disproved' in the truest sense of the word. They are accepted or rejected.

A hypothesis should be clear, concise, logical and specific enough for a reader to understand what the variables are and whom the researcher will be studying. A hypothesis will predict a relationship between variables (for example, difference, greater than, less than, positively, negatively) and, through testing, may or may not allow the relationship to be supported. There are two types of variable – **independent variables** and **dependent variables**. The independent variable is the 'treatment' or 'intervention' variable in the predicted relationship stated in the hypothesis; and the dependent variable is the 'outcome' variable in the relationship. This is commonly known as the 'cause and effect' relationship. There are some examples in Table 7.2.

Table 7.2   *Independent and dependent variables within hypotheses*

More experienced nurses are more likely to express positive comments about the extended role of the nurse than less experienced nurses.

- Level of experience of the nurse is the independent variable.
- Positive comments about the extended role of the nurse is the dependent variable.

Patients who receive a copy of a leaflet about their condition will ask more questions about their care than those who do not receive a leaflet.

- Receiving/not receiving the leaflet is the independent variable.
- Number of questions asked is the dependent variable. Absenteeism is higher in social work students than radiography students.
- Type of student is the independent variable.
- Number of days absent is the dependent variable.

Elderly patients in residential care who experience back massage express greater satisfaction of care than those who do not receive back massage.

- Back massage is the independent variable.
- Satisfaction with care is the dependent variable.

All health and social care practitioners need to be able to recognise research aims, questions and hypotheses when they are reading research reports. The research questions or hypotheses identified should be clearly linked with the original research problem. Not all studies will have a hypothesis. However, where there is one, it should be clearly stated with at least two variables.

KEY POINTS

- Researchable problems have their foundations in practice, literature or an existing theory.
- An early stage in the research process consists of the identification of research aims, questions and hypotheses which must relate to the problem.
- A hypothesis is a statement about a relationship between two or more variables and predicts an expected outcome.

FURTHER READING

Booth, A. (2001). Turning research priorities into answerable research questions. *Health Information and Libraries Journal*, 18 (2), 130–2.
Moule, P. and Goodman, M. (2014). *Nursing research: An introduction* (2nd edn) (pp. 78–101). London: Sage.
Parahoo, K. (2014). *Nursing research: Principles, process and issues* (3rd edn). Basingstoke: Palgrave Macmillan.

WEBSITES

National Institute for Health and Care Excellence: www.nice.org.uk
National Institute for Health Research, RDinfo: http://rdinfo.leeds.ac.uk/Newsletter/Handout.pdf
National Service Frameworks: check websites relevant to topic area, e.g., mental health, diabetes, long-term conditions
Social Care Institute of Excellence: www.scie.org.ukc

8   SAMPLING

LEARNING OUTCOMES

On completion of this chapter the reader should be able to:

- understand definitions of research populations and samples
- identify different sampling strategies that can be employed to select probability and non-probability samples
- consider issues surrounding gaining access to participants
- appreciate the factors that affect sample selection, including sampling criteria and sample size.

KEY CONCEPTS

- non-probability sample
- purposive sample
- stratified sample
- systematic sample
- simple random sample
- snowball sample
- convenience/accidental sample
- representative sample

- target population
- cluster sample
- quota sample
- sample
- sampling
- generalisation
- probability sample
- selection criteria
- bias

INTRODUCTION

Sampling is used in everyday life: for example, when we taste a sip of wine before deciding to buy a bottle or case of it, or at the supermarket we might handle and smell fruit before purchase. Sampling involves the collection of information on which decisions can be based and conclusions drawn. For example, if we liked the taste of the sampled wine we expect to get the same pleasure from bottles containing the same vintage, but could not be certain of our reactions if we purchased a vintage that we had not sampled.

Researchers must collect information from chosen samples, which is then used to make decisions and draw conclusions, just as the purchaser of wine does. The selection of the **sample** is therefore a very important part of the research process. The researcher needs to be confident in drawing conclusions based on the information collected from the chosen sample. Errors in sampling have the potential to invalidate the research findings and render the research unusable.

Before a sample is selected the researcher identifies a **target population**, using techniques, which fall into two main sampling strategies: **probability** and **non-probability sampling**. Prior to describing these strategies, the terms 'target population' and 'sample' must be understood.

TARGET POPULATION

The target population includes the entire membership of the group in which the researcher is interested and from which information can be collected. Such populations might include all students following an undergraduate social work course, all NHS Trust hospitals, or all physiotherapists. Researchers may also collect information from care/clinical situations or documents and in these cases the target population may include all cardio-pulmonary resuscitation attempts, or all completed care-planning documents.

The researcher can assign eligibility criteria to the target population, defining limits within which the target population must fall. For example, the researcher may be interested in the students following a course in therapeutic radiography rather than those following a course in diagnostic radiography. It is therefore necessary to define the target population as students following a course in therapeutic radiography and then select a sample of students who meet this criterion.

The definition of criteria by the researcher facilitates the generalisation (application) of the research findings. In the example given above, research findings could only reliably be applied to students following a course in therapeutic radiography. The degree to which results can be generalised is referred to as **external validity**. External validity can be an important factor in research. However, it should be acknowledged that not all researchers are

interested in achieving external validity. Researchers using a qualitative approach (see Chapter 6) will value the quality of the information collected rather than the ability to generalise the findings
to a larger population.

SAMPLING

It is unlikely that the researcher will be able to collect information
from the entire target population. This would be both time consuming and expensive. The researcher collects information from a
representative sample of the target population, selected by taking
a sample from the target population.

A sample is a portion, or part of, the target population, and is
composed of members (elements or subjects) from which information is collected. In health and social care research the target population may be a patient or client group and the sample will be a
portion of that patient or client group.

The most important feature of sampling is the degree to which
the sample represents the target population. For the sample to
be representative, the members need to reflect the target population in as many ways as possible. For example, how closely do
the characteristics or **variables** such as gender, age, social care
needs, medical diagnosis of the sample, reflect those of the target population?

The reduction of **sampling bias** is also of importance and can
be seen if one part of the target population is over-represented or
under-represented in the sample. For example, if the researcher
was interested in measuring the effectiveness of health promotion strategies and chose to sample people attending health
promotion clinics, it might be argued that those attending the
clinics could have strong views about the benefits of the clinics,
so may be a biased sample.

Limiting the difference between the target population and the
sample is achieved to varying degrees through the application of
accepted sampling techniques in the selection of samples. The two
strategies used to select a sample are probability and non-probability
sampling.

PROBABILITY SAMPLES

Probability sampling involves the use of random selection in
obtaining the sample members. The use of random selection

allows the researcher to state the probability of a member of the target population appearing in the sample. In some cases all members of the target population may have an equal chance of appearing in the sample. Probability sampling limits **sampling errors** and **bias**, increases sample representativeness and gives confidence in the sample. It is therefore the preferred sampling strategy when the researcher is interested in obtaining a representative sample.

Quantitative research designs often employ large probability samples in conducting surveys, experimental and quasi-experimental research (see Chapter 6). It should be noted, however, that qualitative researchers may also use random sampling techniques.

SIMPLE RANDOM SAMPLE

In generating a simple random sample the basic technique of probability sampling is used. When the entire population is known, the use of simple random sampling gives each member of the target population an equal chance of being included in the sample. This occurs through the design of a **sampling frame** in which all members of the target population are represented and from which the sample will be chosen.

The researcher can generate the sampling frame, or an existing sampling frame may be used. If a researcher was interested in sampling qualified and practising nurses and midwives then the register held by the Nursing and Midwifery Council could be accessed and used as a sampling frame.

The use of existing sampling frames can be effective in accessing a sample but a sampling frame needs to be selected appropriately to avoid introducing sampling bias. For example, many market researchers use the telephone directory as a sampling frame. However, it should be acknowledged that as a sampling frame the telephone directory will be an incomplete list of the residents of a community. Not every resident will have a telephone and some of those with a telephone will be ex-directory. The telephone directory will not offer a complete sampling frame and will not therefore facilitate probability sampling. There are a number of approaches that can be used to achieve randomisation with the website www.randomization.com proving a useful resource.

Having generated or obtained an existing sampling frame, the researcher proceeds to randomly select sufficient members from the frame to meet the sample size needed for the study. This can be achieved through the use of a random number table (see Table 8.1). The use of the random number table necessitates numbering the sampling frame members and then selecting from the sampling frame the numbers which correspond with those on the random number table. If selecting a sample of 10 from the random number table of a population of 100 in Table 8.1, the following numbered members would be included in the sample: 03, 35, 11, 98, 74, 20, 23, 61, 32, 30.

Table 8.1   *Random number table*

03	35	11	98	74	20	23	61	32	30
07	09	15	22	21	88	94	90	50	71
84	10	02	91	24	35	47	63	99	04
13	82	31	44	70	65	38	80	92	01
23	33	18	76	97	06	64	53	70	98
17	21	09	05	14	30	31	82	54	56
77	62	02	19	27	48	59	92	71	25
66	04	12	55	42	60	83	24	37	22
05	90	08	69	33	93	57	74	29	10
30	44	74	28	09	67	24	18	99	81
45	89	12	75	65	22	48	21	08	55
78	26	72	03	28	91	36	42	10	89
88	56	23	14	73	54	22	07	52	39
25	78	65	91	63	45	71	01	86	49
67	04	30	05	73	29	96	39	24	49
14	71	27	18	46	28	34	97	24	12
16	48	73	92	45	29	37	19	28	10
13	85	49	37	40	16	72	95	41	08
17	39	73	37	19	91	65	28	76	95
45	42	97	28	02	36	73	95	46	99
77	54	28	16	34	07	16	94	73	54
65	48	27	04	62	48	37	19	21	45
24	91	54	38	18	35	42	87	06	72
06	12	21	26	29	44	79	13	19	46
12	05	43	05	51	10	78	36	58	25
18	25	37	19	54	28	75	53	24	82
96	14	52	75	62	01	99	53	24	42
45	68	24	02	15	73	57	28	27	25
56	81	72	24	04	38	26	78	15	29

In selecting a sample through simple random selection, it is apparent that the researcher cannot intentionally introduce sampling bias. Any bias that occurs will do so by accident, as a result of chance. The likelihood of introducing bias by chance will reduce as the size of the sample selected increases.

It is also apparent that the use of simple random sampling is laborious, and, despite the availability of computer software to generate random numbers, is time consuming. Simple random sampling is used infrequently in sample selection, though the technique of random selection is seen in other probability sampling strategies.

PRACTICE EXAMPLE

Onwujekwe et al. (2009) used simple random sampling strategies in research looking at whether community-based health insurance was an equitable strategy for paying for health care in Nigeria. Community-based health insurance is a form of voluntary health insurance that is increasingly being implemented in Africa. The schemes are funded by annual or more frequent payments and are designed by and for the people. The state of Anambra in Africa has 21 local government areas (LGAS), and the community-based health insurance scheme has been established in 10 of these LGAS, each with a minimum population of 100,000 people. The system was set up to improve the weak health system in the state and was designed to ensure that the populations were being offered equitable services. A publicly owned primary health care centre in each community acts as a focus for the scheme.

To determine whether the scheme did provide equitable health care, two communities were selected from the 10 LGAS. These were selected purposively (see below) as the researchers wanted to work with one site they believed was successful and one they thought might not be. The success or not of the site was measured by the enrolment data in the scheme and the views of the state ministry of health programme officers.

A second stage of simple random sampling was then applied to the purposive sample. All households in the scheme had numbers assigned to them as part of the implementation of the primary health care centre. This numbering was used to select a simple random sample, selecting a predetermined number of participants from the house numbering list. The sample size required was determined through a power calculation, used to ensure the sample size is sufficient to show any difference in statistical significance between the two groups. The numbers for each sample were 455 in the successful site and 516 in the unsuccessful site.

Data were collected from the sample using a pre-tested interviewer administered questionnaire. The head of the household or their representative were interviewed. The results suggested that there was a significant difference in enrolment levels between the two communities, 15.5% in the non-successful and 48.4% in the successful, but that overall there was no inequity in enrolment, both being low. The average premiums were also low and efforts were needed to increase the number of those enrolled. It was suggested that governments and donors should supplement payments made to sustain the health care provision.

This study has therefore used a two-stage sampling strategy. Initially, a purposive sample included two sites that reflected one successful and one unsuccessful. The second stage used a simple random sampling approach to select the participants, using a list of numbers assigned as part of the scheme implementation. This approach limited the influence of the researcher and any sampling biases would have occurred incidentally.

SYSTEMATIC RANDOM SAMPLE

In selecting a systematic random sample a similar technique to that of simple random sampling is employed, as a list of the target population is used to form a sampling frame from which the sample is selected on a systematic basis. In selecting systematically, the researcher may choose, for example, every tenth member on the list or every hundredth member. In this way all members have an equal chance of being selected into the population, provided that all members of the target population are included in the sampling frame and that the sample is not already listed in some sort of systematic way, such as a band 8 nurse through to a band 1–3 employee.

It is possible to select the sample by first calculating the sampling interval for a target population (interval needed between each target member to be selected). To calculate the sampling interval, the researcher would need to know the total number in the target population and the sample size required. For example, if the total target population were 2,000 women who attended an antenatal clinic, and the sample size required were 100 (2,000/100 = 20), then the sample interval is 20. The researcher would select every twentieth woman, following on from the first woman selected from the sampling frame. If the first woman selected was identified as number 2, then women 22, 42, 62, 82, 102, etc. would form the sample.

The sampling technique was used by Assil and Zeidan (2013) in the selection of households to take part in research that examined depression amongst elderly Sudanese aged 60 years or older. The sample included 300 residents of Sudan. Possible participants were identified from three localities, with a total of 50 households being selected to form the final sample. The sampling interval (k) was determined by sample size and took into account the total number of households in each block. The first house was selected randomly and then every kth house anticlockwise was sampled. If the household didn't include an eligible participant then the next house was selected.

Systematic sampling offers a more efficient way of selecting a random sample and the only way that bias can be introduced is by chance. For example, if every kth participant selected by Assil and Zeidan (2013) possessed a particular characteristic, that characteristic would be over-represented in the sample. In this example, every kth participant may have housed an elderly person with a particular mental health issue. A sample composed in this way could be argued to be biased and interpretation of the research findings would need to acknowledge this. As with simple random sampling, the chance of bias would be reduced as the size of the sample increased.

STRATIFIED RANDOM SAMPLE

Selecting a stratified random sample involves the sub-division of the target population into strata, before developing a sampling frame from which a random sample is selected. It is dependent upon the researcher having knowledge of the characteristics or variables of the population, which are important to achieving a representative sample. Sub-division could relate to any variable or characteristic of the target population, such as age, sex, height, weight, ethnic group, socio-economic status, delivery of specific social care, diagnosis, period of admission to hospital or prescribed medications.

Selecting a sample in this way can help achieve a representative sample with a smaller sample size, and so can facilitate more effective use of resources, especially time and money. For example, if a researcher were collecting opinions from physiotherapists about sexual harassment at work, it would be important for the sample to represent the percentage of male and female physiotherapists in the workforce. If the proportion of males were 30% and females were 70%, then a proportionate sample would reflect this.

In some instances the researcher may feel it important to have equal numbers of respondents in the sample to obtain a more balanced view, in this case 50% male and 50% female. This would be a disproportionate sample as it does not represent the male and female composition of the physiotherapist group. The researcher would need to adjust the analysis of any results to compensate for this, by weighting responses.

Stratified sampling enables the researcher to use a smaller sample size to obtain the same measure of representation achieved from a larger simple random sample. It is, therefore, more time and cost effective for the researcher, as using a smaller sample size reduces time spent on data collection and analysis. Sampling error is decreased as variables within the target population, which are critical to the research, are represented through stratification. To achieve this, the researcher has to have knowledge of the target population and, therefore, more effort is required in selecting a sample this way.

PRACTICE EXAMPLE

Vuorenmaa et al. (2013) used a stratified sampling strategy to select participants for a study that evaluated the validity and reliability of the Finnish Family Empowerment Scale (FES) and examined its responsiveness in measuring the empowerment of parents with small children. The scale measures parents' sense of empowerment at the level of family, service delivery and community.

The parents were selected through a stratified sampling strategy using a population information system, the Population Register Centre. All parents included had children aged between 0 and 9 years. The children were stratified into the following age groups: 0–1 years, 2–5 years, 6, 7, 8 and 9 year olds, giving six groupings. The groupings were used to ensure that parents participating would be using different types of child health and education services, such as child health clinics, school health care, day school, pre-school and primary school services. A total of 320 mothers and 320 fathers were identified to evaluate the scale in each of the stratified age groups. A total of 955 parents responded, giving a response rate of 30%. This was a low percentage, raising concerns that perhaps those parents who felt less empowered did not feel able to respond.

(Continued)

(Continued)

Overall, the results suggested the scale was a valid and reliable measure and could be used for measuring empowerment. The use of a stratified sampling strategy ensured that parents using a range of services for children aged 0–9 years were included in evaluating the FES.

CLUSTER SAMPLE

Selecting a cluster sample is a more efficient way of accessing a larger sample than simple or stratified sampling, and is often used to select samples for large-scale surveys, particularly in large geographical areas. Cluster samples can be obtained in situations where a sampling frame cannot be developed using individual members of the target population, as members are not all known to the researcher. This might occur if, for example, the target population were all patients who had recovered from gynaecological surgery.

Cluster sampling can also be referred to as multi-stage sampling, as the researcher selects the sample by following through a number of stages. For example, if the researcher wanted to access patients following gynaecological surgery, a sampling frame composed of organisations treating gynaecological surgical patients would be developed and used to randomly select patients as sample members. The sampling frame might include: regional health authorities, trusts, units, wards and finally patients admitted to the wards. The researcher would first select a regional health authority and then randomly select trusts within that regional health authority. Surgical/gynaecological units would then be selected from the hospitals and gynaecological wards within those units would form the penultimate sample, with patients on the wards being the final sampling frame.

Cluster sampling is more prone to sampling error than simple, stratified and systematic sampling, but offers the researcher a more efficient way of sampling when a large-scale survey is required. As shown in the example above, the technique can also be valuable to the researcher who does not have a sampling frame composed of individual target population members, but is able to commence the sampling process with a sampling frame of organisations or institutions. By following multi-stage sampling techniques, the required sample will be accessed.

NON-PROBABILITY SAMPLES

Non-probability sampling techniques do not use random selection to gather together the sample. Researchers using non-probability sampling will not be able to state the probability of target population members being selected in the sample, as not every member of the target population has a chance of being selected in the sample. Non-probability sampling is more convenient to use, cost effective and can be used to select a research sample when the researcher does not know the membership of the target population. Non-probability sampling techniques include: convenience (accidental) sampling, quota sampling, purposive (judgemental) sampling and snowball sampling. These techniques are often employed in qualitative research designs such as ethnographic, phenomenological, **grounded theory**, exploratory and evaluative designs (see Chapter 6). This said, convenience sampling is commonly used and can be employed in quantitative studies as part of survey or quasi-experimental designs.

CONVENIENCE (ACCIDENTAL) SAMPLING

When employing convenience or accidental sampling techniques the researcher obtains sufficient participants from the local or convenient target population. Participants are included in the sample because they are accessible. For example, a researcher considering the management of social care delivery may select a local sample rather than travelling some distance to obtain a sample.

When employing convenience sampling techniques, it is important for the researcher to acknowledge any limitations in the sample. Convenience sampling is the weakest sampling technique because bias may be introduced into the sample; this is difficult to identify and therefore any effect on the results can be difficult to judge. Bias can result from the over-representation or under-representation of portions of the target population, or from the effect of the researcher sampling locally from a population that is known. Bias may also result if the participants select themselves into the sample, perhaps by responding to market researchers in the street or to advertisements for research participants.

PRACTICE EXAMPLE

Research by Chan and Arthur (2009) entitled 'Nurses' attitudes towards perinatal bereavement care', actually reported a study that included both nurses and midwives in the sample. The nurses were either enrolled or registered nurses and held a midwifery qualification. The study aimed to explore the factors associated with nurses' and midwives' attitudes towards bereavement care at the perinatal stage, such as a stillbirth. The study asked two research questions:

1. What are the nurses' and midwives' attitudes towards perinatal bereavement care?
2. What factors are associated with nurses' and midwives' attitudes towards bereavement care? (2009: 2534)

A power calculation suggested that a sample of 180 was required for the study: 185 nurses/midwives were included, just exceeding the number required. Though the researcher could have used a probability sampling approach, a non-probability convenience sampling strategy was employed. All of the nurses and midwives working in one obstetrics and gynaecology unit were approached. Data was collected using a structured self-completion questionnaire (see Chapter 9). The results suggested that those nurses/midwives with more positive attitudes to hospital policy and training for bereavement care, and who held religious beliefs, were more likely to have a positive attitude to bereavement care.

This research used one local obstetrics and gynaecology unit to obtain the convenience sample of 185 nurses/midwives. The sampling strategy was easy to use, as a local situation and total sample were employed. The sampling strategy would also have helped with effective resource use. The sampling approach does, however, have potential limitations. These were acknowledged by Chan and Arthur, who concluded that the homogeneity of the sample introduced a systematic bias. The fact that the sample were from one hospital, majority Chinese and educated to diploma or below, limits the ability to generalise the results to the entire population of interest.

QUOTA SAMPLING

Selecting a quota sample involves the application of principles which are similar to those used to select a stratified random sample. The researcher uses knowledge of the target population to ensure that certain variables or characteristics of the target population are represented in the sample. The researcher may wish to include any number of variables in the sample: for example, to represent males and females, socio-economic groups, individuals with certain health and social care needs, presence of disease or certain behaviour. By ensuring certain variables are represented in the sample, quota sampling offers a more reliable sampling technique than convenience sampling as it attempts to limit some potential biases.

Robb et al. (2010) used a quota sample when assessing awareness of three National Cancer Screening programmes for breast, cervical and bowel cancer in the UK. The researchers particularly wanted to access the views of ethnic minority populations in the UK. These included: Indian, Pakistani, Bangladeshi, Caribbean, African and Chinese populations. A quota sampling approach ensured all the different populations were represented in the research. In total, 1,500 adults from the six ethnic minority groups completed a questionnaire on their awareness of the screening programmes and undertook face-to-face interviews. The quota numbers for each group needed to be high to achieve the 1,500 total, though in other research these numbers may be lower. It is also worth noting that the quota may relate to a number of characteristics or issues such as gender, socio-economic group, employment or diagnosis.

PURPOSIVE (JUDGEMENTAL) SAMPLING

A purposive sample is selected using the researcher's judgement, with no external objective method being used in sample selection. Reliance on the researcher could be inappropriate and lead to the selection of a biased sample. For example, the researcher might choose sample members who would, it is felt, reflect a certain viewpoint.

Purposive sampling can be a useful sampling technique to employ when the researcher wants to obtain a particular sample, which cannot easily be selected through any other technique.

PRACTICE EXAMPLE

Examples already presented have included purposive sampling as part of their sampling strategy. Chen (2010) used this sampling approach alone, as part of recent research. The research aimed to explore the

(Continued)

(Continued)

perceived barriers older adults residing in long-term care institutions experience in taking regular physical activity. A purposive sampling strategy was used to recruit older adults who needed to meet inclusion criteria:

1. Be 65 years of age or older.
2. Not engaging in any regular physical exercise.
3. Resident in a nursing home for at least six months.
4. No obvious cognitive and mental impairment.
5. Able to communicate.

The sample were purposively selected from six nursing homes located in two areas in Taiwan. The mean age of the participants was 78.5 years, with a range of 65–90 years. In total, 90 people were interviewed. The results suggested that barriers to physical activity included physical health problems, fear of falls or injury, previous sedentary lifestyle, lack of understanding about the importance of exercise and environmental factors that prohibited exercise.

   The researcher needed to work with a sample of older adults, who would be able to give consent and answer open-ended questions. They also needed to be residents in long-term care institutions and not taking part in any regular exercise. Using a purposive sample of nursing homes enabled Chen to select participants who met the inclusion criteria. There are some limitations to this sampling strategy as it relies on the researcher's judgement; however, sample site selection would have been guided by the research aim and the set sampling criteria.

SNOWBALL SAMPLING

A **snowball sample** can be a useful technique for selecting a 'hidden' sample group, such as the homeless. Snowball sampling is based on the assumption that people with like characteristics, behaviours or interests, form associations, and it is this relationship which the researcher uses to select a sample. For example, access to a group of experts can be gained by approaching one expert who recommends possible further respondents. Access to the homeless, drug abusers and alcoholics can be obtained through one group member, who recommends further sample members and thus a self-generating sample is facilitated. Biases may be introduced as the sample is not independently selected and the sample could perpetuate particular traits. However, it can be a useful way of selecting a sample from marginalised groups.

PRACTICE EXAMPLE

A qualitative study conducted by Merrell et al. (2006) included purposive and snowball sampling as part of its design. The research aimed to 'identify the health and social care needs of Bangladeshi carers, who were caring for a dependent relative' (2006: 198). Access to the sample was a challenge for the researchers, largely because the population is hidden. Bangladeshi carers didn't use local voluntary or statutory carer groups that might have provided a forum for easier access. To overcome the challenge, the researchers recruited a research assistant from the Bangladeshi community to gain access through a combined strategy of purposive and snowball sampling. The assistant used purposive sampling to identify an initial carer, who was then used to start a snowball sampling approach. Each carer interviewed was asked to nominate another for interview until the researcher achieved a sample of 20. Chen acknowledges the limitations of this approach, noting that snowball sampling can lead to the recruitment of participants from similar backgrounds.

It is clear that when a sample is hidden, as in this case, snowball sampling can be used to access an appropriate sample. The other non-probability sampling approaches discussed in this chapter can only be used if the sample is easily identifiable by the researcher. Fortunately, Chen had links with one Bangladeshi carer and was able to use this participant, identified through purposive sampling, to identify another carer who became the first of 19 accessed through snowball sampling. Despite its limitations, the approach can be the only strategy available to researchers working with certain populations.

ISSUES RELATING TO SAMPLE SIZE

There are no hard and fast rules governing the selection of sample size. The choice of the sample, using the techniques described in this chapter, is of greater importance than the choice of a particular sample size. However, a technique known as power analysis can be applied to estimate an appropriate sample size. This can be applied particularly in quantitative studies, when certain statistical tests are applied to the results and when the generalisation of results to a wider population is of importance. The discussion of power analysis is beyond the scope of this introductory text, but can be found in Burns and Grove (2013), included as further reading on the following page.

It is generally accepted that a larger probability sample will give greater accuracy to the results, as the effect of over-representation or under-representation is reduced as the sample size increases. Non-probability samples may use a smaller sample size more effectively, particularly if the researcher is interested in the value of the quality of the information collected (qualitative approach), rather than the quantity of information which could be gathered (quantitative approach). Whichever sampling technique is used, the representative nature of the sample is of greater importance than the size.

GAINING ACCESS TO SUBJECTS

In order to undertake research it is necessary to gain access to the sources of data. In health and social care research these are generally people, but sources could also be records, documents or personally related data. Sometimes the sources of the data will be 'protected' and the researcher may need to negotiate carefully with people in powerful positions, or with institutions. The term **gatekeeper** is often used to describe people who are attempting to safeguard the interests of others. These could, for example, be teachers protecting students on a course, or managers protecting employees. When research is taking place in health or social care settings, such as clinics or wards, the researcher will need to gain permission from key individuals such as clinical managers. If patients, and in many cases staff, are involved, the proposed research will need to meet **research governance** requirements and be considered by a local **Research Ethics Committee** (see Chapter 4). Academics and health care students may also need to apply to their university ethics committee.

Acquiring permission or consent of the subjects is also an important factor in gaining access. This can be particularly difficult when the research is covert, such as **participant observation** studies.

Many ethical issues need to be considered by the researcher, such as deception, concealment and not gaining consent from subjects who clearly need to be protected. Dealing with gatekeepers and negotiating access is a responsibility that the researchers must take seriously in order to protect research integrity. When reading research critically, health and social care professionals must consider ways that the researcher may have negotiated this process.

KEY POINTS

- Researchers must collect information from chosen samples.
- The researcher selects a sample from the target population.
- Sampling bias can occur if one element of the target population is over- or under-represented.
- The two overall strategies used to select a sample are probability and non-probability sampling.
- There are no hard and fast rules about the size of sample needed to support research, though the use of statistical tests in quantitative studies may dictate sample size.

FURTHER READING

Alston, M. and Bowles, W. (2012). *Research for social workers: An introduction to methods* (3rd edn). London: Routledge.
Burns, N. and Grove, S. (2013). *The practice of nursing research: Appraisal, synthesis and generation of evidence* (7th edn). St Louis, MO: Saunders Elsevier.
Hicks, C. (2009). *Research methods for clinical therapists: Applied project design and analysis* (6th edn). Edinburgh: Churchill Livingstone.
Moule, P. and Goodman, M. (2014). *Nursing research: An introduction* (2nd edn). London: Sage.

WEBSITES

National Cancer Institute, discussion on randomisation: www.cancer.gov/clinical trials/understanding/what-is-randomization
Randomization website: www.randomization.com

9 UNDERSTANDING DATA COLLECTION TECHNIQUES

LEARNING OUTCOMES

On completion of this chapter the reader should be able to:

- appreciate the need for reliable and valid data collection methods in health and social care research
- identify the main data collection techniques used in health and social care research
- understand the need to choose data collection techniques appropriate to the research approach and design
- evaluate the advantages and disadvantages of different measuring instruments.

KEY CONCEPTS

- documentary evidence
- non-participant observer
- observation schedule
- repertory grid
- questionnaire
- observation
- Visual Analogue Scale
- interview
- rigour
- participant observer
- rating scale
- trustworthiness
- vignettes
- Likert scale
- secondary data collection
- psychological measures
- physiological measures
- reliability
- validity
- triangulation

INTRODUCTION

Research information can be collected in many ways. The researcher's choice of data collection instrument is influenced by the research approach (qualitative or quantitative) and the research questions to be addressed. The researcher must be confident that the instrument or instruments used will collect information relevant to the research question, and support the research approach taken.

RELIABILITY AND VALIDITY

The researcher is also concerned about the **reliability** and **validity** of the data collection method used. Both reliability and validity are important as they afford credibility to the data collection tool and subsequent research findings. A valid and reliable instrument will measure what it is expected to measure, and be consistent or dependable in measuring what it is designed to measure (Moule and Goodman, 2014). For example, the tympanic thermometer is seen as a valid and reliable way of measuring temperature. Unless broken it will measure a patient's temperature when the principles of correct temperature taking are followed, and will measure every patient's temperature in the same way.

It should be remembered that there is always room for error in measurement. For example, if the principles of correct temperature taking using a tympanic thermometer are not followed the thermometer may record an abnormally high or low temperature that will not reflect the patient's true temperature. Data collection is therefore open to some inconsistency. Any inconsistency should be acknowledged by the researcher and may lead to the adoption of research practices that will enhance reliability, such as using several data collection methods. If a data collection instrument is not, however, a valid measure, and is not recording what it is expected to, then the researcher must look to alternative measuring tools.

ESTABLISHING TRUSTWORTHINESS

Qualitative research methods are essentially different to quantitative methods and there is a need to evaluate qualitative methods against different and appropriate criteria. Lincoln and Guba (1985) present specific steps that can be taken to try to ensure rigour and **trustworthiness** in qualitative research: ensuring credibility, transferability, dependability and confirmability. To establish trustworthiness data must be auditable through checking that the interpretations are credible. The credibility of data is improved through long engagement with the respondents or **triangulation** (using three or more methods) of data collection. 'Thick' description (thorough description of the research setting and process) can enable the reader to determine how transferable the results may be to another setting. An audit trail of the research assists in establishing the dependability of the research and confirmability, through the inclusion of information such as the presentation of **raw data** and an explanation of **data analysis** processes.

The most commonly used data collection instruments will be discussed in this chapter. They include: physiological and psychological measures, measurement scales, **questionnaires**, **interviews**, **observations** and documentary sources. The chapter will not discuss the ways in which any information collected through measurement could be analysed, as this is fully considered in Chapter 10.

PHYSIOLOGICAL AND PSYCHOLOGICAL MEASURES

Both physiological and psychological measures are important to health and social care practice. Both types of measures are used on a day-to-day basis to record patient and client information. Many of these measures provide valuable information for the health and social care team, and, as valid and reliable measuring tools, they are often used by researchers. There are a variety of measuring instruments available to the researcher, including electronic tools.

The range of valid and reliable physiological measures available is too vast to list. Examples include: digital blood pressure monitors; measurements of nerve impulses; digital and tympanic thermometers that record temperature; strip tests that indicate urine composition; and biochemical tests that measure blood composition.

Many of these measures have been employed in the collection of research information and have been the subject of research that has considered the reliability of temperature recording tools. For example, Farnell et al. (2005) assessed the accuracy and reliability of two non-invasive methods of temperature measurement in an intensive care environment. One hundred and sixty temperature sets from 25 adults were recorded using chemical (Tempa Dot™) and tympanic thermometers (Genius™ First Temp M3000A) and compared against the gold standard pulmonary artery catheter. The findings suggested the chemical thermometer was more accurate and reliable when compared with the tympanic thermometer. However, compared with the pulmonary artery catheter both methods gave erroneous recordings.

There are many psychological measures available to the researcher. For example, the State Trait Anxiety Inventory measures anxiety that increases as a result of threat (state anxiety), and anxiety that is an inherent part of the person's personality (trait anxiety). The measure offers a useful way of recording anxiety level and it has been used by many researchers.

PRACTICE EXAMPLE

A State Trait Anxiety Inventory (STAI) was used in research conducted by Comeaux and Steele-Moses (2013). The quasi-experimental design (see Chapter 6) determined whether music therapy was an effective adjunct to standard treatment for post-operative pain. The control group received standard treatment and the intervention group received complimentary music therapy, being provided with pre-programmed MP3 players, in addition to the standard treatment. The STAI was completed before the treatment and one day after the intervention was in place. Prior to the intervention both groups were matched in their levels of state and trait anxiety, pain and noise perception. However, following treatment the pain perception and noise perception measures showed a significant difference, whereas there was no change in the state anxiety ($p = 0.711$). The findings suggest that the use of music therapy decreases noise and pain perception, but fails to have any effect on state anxiety.

This study provides an example of the use of STAI to measure the levels of anxiety. The STAI can be used in any research where changes in anxiety levels are an important outcome measure.

The researcher needs to select the most appropriate physiological and psychological instruments to use in the research, which should be both valid and reliable measures. In preparation for data collection, the functioning and availability of equipment will need to be considered. Training in data collection methods, including use of equipment, must be complete before data collection can commence.

MEASUREMENT SCALES

Polit and Beck (2014) suggest that a scale is a device which allows the assignment of numerical scores to a continuum measuring attributes, such as the scale that measures weight, the scale that measures shoe size or the scale that records height. Many scales are used generally in society. Within health and social care, scales are used to measure specific phenomena and are important to daily practice. Such scales may, for example, measure pain response, nutritional status, risk of pressure sore development, and client satisfaction.

There are many valid and reliable scales available for use in health and social care research (Bowling, 2009), many of which are used in practice. The researcher may be able to select existing scales that will achieve the desired research outcome, provided copyright is sought. This overcomes validity and reliability issues that can arise when designing a new measuring scale, which would need to be tried and tested before use.

Scales may be the sole data collection instrument used by the researcher, or may be one of many data collection tools employed. Scales may also be included within the design of questionnaires (see later). Within this chapter the rating scale, **Likert scale** and **Visual Analogue Scale**, **repertory grid** and **vignettes** are considered.

Rating scales are used to attribute a numerical score to an assessment or judgement (Brace, 2013). The respondent is asked a question and then is guided to select from a series of numbered statements the one that reflects their assessment or judgement. The rating scale can be used to rate client satisfaction with the quality of care received. The client may be asked, for example, to assess the quality of information giving, and grade the information given in relation to a scale of 0–5, with 0 being unsatisfactory and 5 being completely satisfactory.

The scale may be used for example, in gathering information from elderly residents about their care environment, as in Figure 9.1.

Burns and Grove (2013) suggest rating scales can be easy to generate, and offer a useful form of measurement provided the end statements are not so extreme as to affect their selection. The scales are, however, crude measures, and the information generated in this way is limited. In the example above, the attitude of staff may be rated in relation to one poor experience or one very positive experience; in other words, the client's response can be swayed by one event, rather than reflecting a general impression.

The Likert scale is a commonly used scale. Named after psychologist Rensis Likert, it is used to obtain attitude or opinion to ten or more statements. The scale is a more refined tool that forces the respondent to give their opinion on a series of statements, indicating whether they: strongly disagree, disagree, are neutral or unsure, agree, or strongly agree. Usually the scale includes five values, to which numerical scores can be ascribed. More commonly, a high score (5) is achieved by agreement with a positively worded statement and disagreement with a negative statement (Polit and Beck, 2014). Figure 9.2 gives an example of this.

Please rate from 1 (low) – 10 (high), the following statements in relation to your care:	
	Rating
1 Quietness during the day	( )
2 Quietness during the night	( )
3 Choice of food	( )
4 Heating	( )
5 Bathroom facilities	( )
6 Attitude of staff	( )
7 Provision of social facilities	( )
8 Cleanliness of the residence	( )
9 Comfort of the bed	( )

Figure 9.1   *Example of a rating scale*

	Strongly agree	Agree	Neutral	Disagree	Strongly disagree	Score
1 Children behaving badly benefit from individual attention	✓					5
2 Children behaving badly do not benefit from individual attention	✓					1

Figure 9.2   *An example of a Likert scale used to measure attitude to discipline in children*

In Figure 9.2, the response to statement one receives a score of 5, as the respondent strongly agrees with a positive statement. If the respondent had strongly disagreed with the positive statement, a score of 1 would be allocated. The response to statement two receives a score of 1, as the respondent has strongly agreed to a negative statement. To strongly disagree with this statement would achieve a score of 5.

The scale should be composed of equal numbers of negative and positive statements. If the scale included only positive statements, it would be easy for the respondent to select only positive responses, agreeing with all the statements without thought. There is the potential for respondents to continually choose neutral responses and thus give no impression of attitude or opinion. Respondents might also give the response that meets current 'no smacking' thinking.

PRACTICE EXAMPLE

Gharaibeh and Mater (2009) conducted a study to identify young Syrian adults' knowledge, perceptions and attitudes to premarital testing for the risk of potential genetic disorders. In total 942 students completed a questionnaire that consisted of 42 items and was scored using a Likert scale (1 = strongly disagree, 2 = disagree, 3 = uncertain, 4 = agree, 5 = strongly agree). A pilot study tested the reliability of the questionnaire, and it achieved a high reliability coefficient of 0.83, meaning the scale was likely to be a reliable tool for collecting the data required. Within the questionnaire there were groups of items related to attitudes and perceptions. The scoring for each item was calculated based on the mean (average) score for the student's item responses. A score of 3.5 or higher was viewed as high knowledge or positive perception and attitude.

The Likert scale developed was able to identify knowledge, attitude and perception of the students in relation to a sensitive issue and enabled the researchers to gather a large amount of data from one university site in a short space of time. The overall results showed that whilst the students were knowledgeable about premarital testing, there were some gaps in their knowledge and they did have mixed attitudes and perceptions, some being positive and some negative.

Other methods of assessing attitudes include repertory grids and vignettes. The repertory grid is a technique used by the researcher to elicit an individual's constructs (perceptions) concerning specific issues through deep exploration of the individual's perceptions, expressed in their own words. Further explanations of the technique can be seen in Bowling (2009).

Vignettes are short descriptions of a topic of interest, event, situation, scenario or case history, which are presented to respondents with a series of structured questions. Vignettes are most commonly written descriptions, though can be video clips online that are used to gain information about the respondent's perceptions, opinions or knowledge about a situation (Bowling, 2009; Polit and Beck, 2014).

PRACTICE EXAMPLE

McCrow et al. (2013) developed and reviewed five vignettes for use in the education of nurses. Five vignettes were developed that depicted older people with a range of cognitive impairments, such as dementia and delirium. The accuracy and reliability of the vignettes was established through a process of formal review. This involved 19 international experts from the field reviewing the content for accuracy and suggesting revisions. This process was structured around the completion of an expert review questionnaire.

The use of vignettes is increasing within research that seeks to measure learning and practice change. They provide a written simulation of real patients where questions are developed to ascertain the practitioner's ability to assess, implement and evaluate care of a patient. Expert advice is required in the generation of the vignette and marking criteria.

The Visual Analogue Scale is a vertical or horizontal line, measuring 0–100 mm, with each millimetre representing a numerical score (Polit and Beck, 2014). The end points of the scale symbolise extreme values, with the line denoting all values between. The measurement of pain experience can be achieved using a scale with end points representing unbearable pain and no pain, with all other pain experiences being found along the scale. When using the scale, the patient marks along the line the point, which they feel represents their current pain response (see Figure 9.3).

In constructing the scale, the values used to identify the end points need consideration, as they need to reflect extremes.

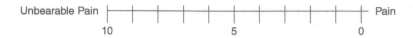

Figure 9.3   *Visual Analogue Scale*

There may also be potential difficulties in obtaining a true response. In the example above, patients may be reluctant to admit to having unbearable pain.

PRACTICE EXAMPLE

The Visual Analogue Scale (VAS) is often used by researchers to measure symptoms such as pain experience. Used in this way by Heneweer et al. (2010), the VAS of a 100 mm line was used to measure pain experience in 69 patients with sub-acute lower back pain. Measurements with the VAS were taken at two, four, eight and twelve weeks. The tool provided a reliable measure of pain intensity that was self-administered. It enabled the researchers to look at pain experience as part of a series of measures. The tool is easily developed, has high reliability and is easily used.

In selecting measurement scales the researcher will need to know which scales are available and feel confident that the scales used will be sensitive enough to obtain the responses required. In addition, the researcher will need to know that the scales are valid and reliable measures.

QUESTIONNAIRES

The questionnaire is the most frequently used data collection instrument. It is composed of a series of written questions which usually require written responses. The questionnaire can be used to collect information that is amenable to statistical analysis, and it can therefore be used to collect data in quantitative studies.

The questionnaire offers the researcher flexibility in delivery as it can be administered by hand to individuals, to groups of people, or can be posted or emailed to reach a large number of people across a wide geographical area. It is often, therefore, the data collection instrument chosen for use in surveys. In addition, the questionnaire can be completed anonymously, which can be of value in research studies where honest opinion is sought, or in situations of unequal researcher and respondent status. For example, questionnaires can be useful in collecting information from service users as part of auditing the quality of care being delivered by a particular service or professional.

While reviewing the literature, the researcher may identify a questionnaire that would be an appropriate tool for use in the research study. With the original author's consent, it would be possible to use the same or slightly modified instrument and thus save valuable time in questionnaire generation.

The construction of a new questionnaire requires skill and can be time consuming. The questionnaire must include questions that will elicit responses needed to address the research question. This process requires skill and knowledge in questionnaire design. In addition, the researcher must establish the validity and reliability of the instrument, using the instrument to collect data, perhaps as part of a **pilot study** (see Chapter 3).

When formulating a questionnaire, the researcher makes decisions about its structure and layout. The main types of question included are open or closed. Open questions require a response of one or more words or sentences. For example, the question, 'In your own words, describe what social care is', would probably be answered in a few sentences. Closed questions are structured to offer the respondent a choice of answers. The scales discussed earlier might be used within this structure. An example of a closed question is seen in Figure 9.4.

Questions should not be leading, such as, 'You don't support this new idea, do you?', nor should they be value laden or ask more than one question at a time. One example of this is the commonly used question, 'Do you want a cup of tea and do you want a biscuit?', which is in fact asking two questions at once. The organisation of questions is also important. Asking sensitive questions at the beginning of the questionnaire can adversely affect response rates. It is usual to establish personal details, and ask general questions first, before moving on to more specific and directed questions. The researcher will also need to allow sufficient space to enable the respondent to give full answers. The development of information technologies has meant that some researchers are using the internet or email to deliver questionnaires. For example, Cunningham et al. (2009) used a computerised questionnaire placed in emergency departments to obtain feedback from young adults on alcohol use. Other researchers collect data using electronic devices such as Personal Digital Assistants and mobile phones.

Please tick the appropriate response:

1 Sex

    Male   ( )01

    Female   ( )02

2 Length of experience in professional role

    1–3 years   ( )01

    4–6 years   ( )02

    7–10 years   ( )03

    11–15 years   ( )04

    16–20 years   ( )05

    20+ years   ( )06

Figure 9.4 *An example of closed questions with coded responses*

Instructions for completion of the questionnaire need to be clear, particularly as the researcher is often not available to clarify any queries. The researcher should include a covering letter of introduction, in which response deadlines may be set and incentives may be offered. It is not uncommon for researchers to offer material reward to those completing a questionnaire.

As part of questionnaire construction the researcher must consider data analysis. Closed questions might be coded, as shown in Figure 9.4. In question 1, the codes 01 and 02 relate to the sex of the respondents. These codes would be used to prepare the data for analysis. Analysis of open questions would be concerned with identifying specific content, and thus forms part of **content analysis**, which is discussed as part of data analysis in Chapter 10.

The potential benefits of using a questionnaire to collect research data relate to the effective use of researcher time, reduced costs, access to a world-wide sample, access to a large **sample** at one time, **anonymity**, and reduced researcher **bias**. The potential drawbacks can include difficulties in questionnaire construction and exclusion of certain sample groups, such as children and those with language or learning difficulties. There is the potential to alienate certain groups from the research if a barrier such as availability of questionnaires in different languages is not considered. Furthermore, the researcher may receive unexpected responses but is unable to pursue these further as the individual respondents are not identified.

The expected respondent may not complete the questionnaire, and additional disadvantages might include unsatisfactory completion, rendering the questionnaire useless and spoilt. Response rates can be poor, with mailed questionnaires often achieving a 25–30% response (Burns and Grove, 2013). If a response of less than 50% is achieved, the representativeness of the sample can be called into question (Burns and Grove, 2013).

PRACTICE EXAMPLE

A postal questionnaire used by Damery et al. (2010) aimed at investigating GP attitudes to colorectal cancer screening yielded a low response rate. Of the 3,191 GPS surveyed, there were 960 returned responses that could be used by the researchers. One reminder was sent out to respondents, a process that can increase return levels. The respondents were also provided with a freepost envelope for return. This can also help increase questionnaire return rates. Despite the use of return freepost envelopes and a reminder, the overall response rate was 30.7%. This was disappointingly low, though just exceeds the percentage return that Burns and Grove (2013) suggest is often seen when postal questionnaires are used. The researchers report that they didn't offer an incentive to encourage completion. This approach can be used to help completion rates and the incentives offered could include offering entry to a free prize draw or supplying book or other tokens when completed surveys are returned.

When response appears low, it is accepted that researchers will follow up the sample with reminders, either by post or email. Response to postal questionnaires is also aided by providing stamped and addressed reply envelopes, as well as including reply dates as part of an introductory letter, as mentioned earlier. If they have been administered by hand, the researcher might collect the questionnaires or organise a collection point, which will aid response.

INTERVIEWS

Interviews are the second most frequently used data collection technique, and involve the collection of information by verbal communication. Interviews can be conducted on an individual basis either face-to-face or over the telephone, or within a group setting. The interview can be used in qualitative research, to collect in-depth information from which theory can be generated. An interview may also form part of a quantitative design, when a structured interview schedule is used.

The interview schedule is constructed using many of the principles of questionnaire design (see earlier) and includes a list of questions to be posed. The researcher works systematically through the schedule, recording responses. This format can be used in a face-to-face interview or in a telephone interview.

Face-to-face interviews can be less structured, with the researcher identifying one or more key questions that can give some organisation to the interview. The researcher, ultimately allowing the respondent to give direction to the interview, can explore individual responses to the questions. This open design can yield in-depth information about people's opinions, attitudes and feelings, and can be used in individual or group interviews.

The focus group is composed of 6 to 12 members of differing opinion, who meet to discuss research issues (Bowling, 2009). The group discussion can last from one to three hours and is based on outline questions generated through **literature review**. The facilitator poses the questions or statements and records the group discussion. The focus group can provide a useful forum for discussing a range of topics, offering the researcher rich data from which further research questions can be generated.

The researcher must decide which interview design will enable the collection of data needed to address the research question. Questions used in an interview must be constructed following the principles of question formation (see Questionnaires earlier in this chapter). In particular the content of questions and the organisation of questions need consideration.

As interviews necessitate verbal interaction, the researcher needs to consider how to gain access to the sample, making arrangements to conduct interviews at a time convenient to the respondent. The researcher must also consider the duration of the interview, with 45 minutes being a realistic maximum participation time. These points would apply if the interview were conducted over the telephone or face-to-face. The researcher needs a suitable environment for the interview, with privacy and quietness being important considerations.

The recording of an interview may or may not involve the use of technology. Written recording of interviewee responses is often used and can be preferred by respondents who may object to being electronically recorded. However, the researcher might find it useful to record an interview on disc or videotape. This facilitates analysis of content as the researcher can listen to the interview several times and, if it has been videoed, may be able to identify non-verbal communication more easily. Audio recordings can be transcribed more readily, which will also aid analysis. The researcher may ask a second person to view or listen to recordings, to help with the analysis process. In obtaining a second viewpoint, the researcher may be alerted to new information that had been overlooked, and may be forced to re-examine their perceptions of the interview, which helps validate the findings, thus improving analysis.

Interviewing is a skill that is often presumed to be innate. It is, however, a skill that needs developing, as is depicted by many experienced television interviewers. The researcher is therefore likely to use the pilot study to test the interview schedule or questions, as well as to develop interviewing skills. The interviewer must consider habits, such as nodding or smiling, used in asking questions as the interviewee might identify these as cues to the sort of response that is wanted. The interviewer has the potential to bias the results in many ways, such as through non-verbal and verbal cues, and by the nature of the relationship with the respondent. A researcher in a perceived position of power may not receive true responses, and a researcher seen to be of lower status than the respondent may be dealt with in a dismissive way by the interviewee.

Guaranteeing anonymity might overcome some of the difficulties encountered when trying to gain truthful information from respondents. There are special considerations when using vulnerable groups, such as those with mental health problems, as the research sample. The researcher must be confident that the respondents are enabled to divulge their true feelings and opinions, and acknowledge that the results may be affected by the person's dependency or vulnerability.

Interviews provide a flexible data collection tool, which can allow the researcher to explore pertinent issues raised during the course of the interview. The interview can provide detailed information, and may also be useful in collecting data from groups unable to respond to a questionnaire, such as children.

The organisation of interviews requires thought. Interviews are also time consuming, with each interview possibly taking about 45 minutes, 30 minutes of which is spent collecting data. Interviewer bias and the researcher–respondent relationship may affect the quality of the information collected.

PRACTICE EXAMPLE

A mixture of telephone interviews and focus groups was used as the main method of data collection by Kelly and Nisker (2010). Exploring whether final year medical students felt prepared to address end-of-life issues, they recorded conversations over the telephone with 20 participants and ran a focus group with five. The format of data collection was the same, with key prompt questions that explored experiences of death and coping strategies. The data was transcribed verbatim and analysed using a grounded theory approach (see Chapter 6). Detail isn't provided as to the length of data collection, though the guide questions suggest the focus group is unlikely to have been lengthy, and normally telephone interviews are shorter than face-to-face interactions. The focus group is a reasonable size, though it could have been larger had more students elected to participate in this way. The fact that the researchers offered different ways for participants to engage probably aided the final sample size, particularly in this case where the sample group have pressured workloads and limited time for engagement.

OBSERVATIONS

Observational studies collect information from the observation of behaviours or events. Information collected in this way is not often numerical, but is a written record of the researcher's interpretation of events, and is therefore a method that is employed mostly in qualitative research. Observational studies can record the complexity of health and social care, which may not easily be measured using any self-reporting methods, such as interviews and questionnaires. However, there are a number of ethical issues associated with this research method, requiring the researcher to operate in an open way adopting an 'overt role' as either participant or non-participant observer.

The participant observer is part of the situation under observation and needs to maintain a clinical role whilst recording data, which may prove problematic. The non-participant observer would be identified as a researcher, perhaps sitting in a sports centre observing the use of the swimming facilities. The researcher would need some insight and knowledge of the events observed to interpret observations made. The researcher assuming anonparticipant role may use more structured data collection tools, such as an observation schedule. The schedule would be predetermined, allowing recording of events under observation in a structured way. For example, the schedule might record verbal interactions with a group of patients on the ward. This would necessitate recording with whom the interactions are made, and the time taken to complete conversation. The researcher would use codes to identify all possible personnel involved to facilitate easy recording. The end result might appear as in Figure 9.5.

Time/Patient	Alan	Perry	Miles	David	Ken
0900 hours	A,D	N	C	/	L
0905	/	N	M	I	L
0910	/	N	M	/	L
0915	G,E,F,D	N	B,C	/	L
0920	E,D	G,E,F,D	/	/	L
0925	E,D	/	G,E,F,D	O	N

Key

A = health care assistant	I = ward clerk
B = student nurse	J = relatives
C = staff nurse	K = other patients
D = sister/charge nurse	L = dietician
E = house officer	M = physiotherapist
F = registrar	N = occupational therapist
G = consultant	O = social worker
H = domestic	P = other

Figure 9.5   *An example of an observation schedule used to record verbal interaction with patients*

To achieve consistency in measurement, there needs to be parity in the recording and interpretation of information. This can be achieved using recording techniques and through training the observer. In some instances it may be useful to have more than one observer to overcome difficulties with observer reliability and bias.

Recording information gained through observation can pose difficulty for the researcher. A non-participant observer might use an observation schedule, as discussed earlier, or a one-way mirror, or may even record events on video for later analysis. The participant observer needs to either memorise events or find some way of recording field notes.

Access to the sample can also be more problematic. The researcher must organise access to the environment and needs to consider time-management, as observations may take from days to weeks or months. There are many issues surrounding the potential effects observational studies may have on the sample, as such studies can be more invasive and obtrusive.

Observations can be problematic for the participants, requiring changes to accommodate either researcher or data collection instruments. The constant presence of researchers or data collection instruments may also affect the quality of observation. The 'hawthorne effect' is a well-documented account of the effect of researcher presence on the research outcomes. To measure the hawthorne effect, researchers, considering how to increase productivity at an electrical plant, made recommendations based on the increase in productivity seen during their research, which changed heating, light and rest time. These recommendations were adopted by the managers, who then saw production fall. Researcher presence had therefore led to a temporary increase in production. The researcher can, therefore, introduce bias to the observations, by affecting the events observed.

Recording the data relates to the observer role adopted. The non-participant observer may use an observation schedule and find concentration on events easier than the participant observer. There may, however, be ethical dilemmas for the researcher to cope with. For example, if a nurse researcher is recording events in a ward area when a cardiac arrest occurs, there may be personal dilemma between continuing the observer role and the need to react as a nurse to the situation. This is sometimes called the 'dual role' of researcher/practitioner.

The participant observer may have difficulties recording information, though the information gained may be more insightful. Additional problems may arise if the researcher becomes subsumed into the culture, which might affect their objective interpretation of the situation.

Observational studies can provide an in-depth understanding of events, particularly if the researcher has experienced the subject of the research. Often observation may be the only technique available to collect the information needed. However, observational methods rely on the researcher's perceptions and interpretations of events, and are therefore open to individual bias. There are also ethical and organisational issues to consider, including access, recording data, role adoption and management of time. Observations can offer the researcher information which might not be obtained using self-reporting techniques, and this is particularly evident when considering behaviour and events.

PRACTICE EXAMPLE

Eriksson et al. (2010) used observations when trying to interpret the interplay between the critically ill patient and their next of kin in an intensive care environment. Ten patients were included in the study, who met a set of selection criteria that included: ≤ 18 years old; reason for admission was serious illness or acute illness; they were in the intensive care environment for ≥ 48 hours; they were ventilated for ≥ 24 hours; and were visited at least once by next of kin. In total 24 visits made by relatives were observed. The patients were cared for by two nurses in a two-roomed bay and visiting was open and around the clock. Family members provided informed consent prior to the study, with consent being sought from the patients after the treatment period.

Data was collected through non-participant observations, completed by the lead researcher, who was involved in the administration and education for the intensive care unit, but not the hands-on care delivery. The observations focused on the interplay between the patients and relatives, recorded during a maximum period of two hours. Observations were not structured. Observations were recorded along with reflective notes. The transcription of the interaction was recorded and analysed by considering the text as a script for a play with a discussion of the scene, actors and plot.

The findings suggested the intensive care environment prohibited interplay as it was designed for medical and technical use rather than promoting healing.

The non-participatory approach taken meant that the observer was able to concentrate on recording the interactions between the patients and relatives. Some of the potential difficulties of having a dual role of researcher and professional were also avoided, as the researcher had no role related to care delivery on the unit. Sometimes if researchers are part of the care delivery team, but have an observer role, there are tensions in trying to maintain observations if there is a need for care delivery. There is, however, the potential for the

(Continued)

(Continued)

'hawthorne effect' as the researcher presence could have affected the interactions. However, conducting the observations for two-hour periods, rather than shorter sessions, might have lessened the impact of this.

Observational research such as this is time consuming and therefore potentially resource intensive, which has an impact on funding levels. Additionally, there are potential ethical issues if the observer is covert (hidden), and even if they are known, as in this case, prolonged observation can be intrusive. The effect of intrusion was minimised in this case by limiting the observation periods to two hours in length. Technology is used by some researchers (video or digital recording) to reduce some of the impact of cost and intrusion.

DOCUMENTARY EVIDENCE

Existing documents are a rich source of research information that form part of **secondary data** collection techniques. Researchers may be able to access and interpret many health and social care documents, such as case notes, census data, care pathways, minutes of committee meetings, policy papers and letters. This facilitates analysis of existing material that has been collected for a purpose other than research, which is identified as secondary data.

Other types of documentary evidence have been used in many research studies. For example, Moloney et al. (2009) explored the feasibility and acceptability of an internet-based diary to obtain acceptable completion rates of diaries, in research looking at migraine sufferers. Diaries are widely used to record the incidence of headaches, but this was the first time an internet-based diary had been used. The diaries were completed over a four-month period by 77 participants. The researchers concluded the internet-based diaries were an acceptable data collection tool, which enabled participation across a geographically spread population. It should be noted, however, that only those with internet access can be recruited.

The increased recording of documentary information in health care is likely to provide greater impetus for its use in research. Secondary data sources are likely to gain popularity in the research field as data recording improves, and the reduced costs and time involved in using existing documentary sources will also be factors affecting their future use (Bowling, 2009).

Other considerations in using documentary evidence relate to researcher bias, which may be reduced if someone else has completed the initial recording of information. However, relying on data collected by others can bring its own problems, as when, for instance, records are rendered useless because of initial recording problems. Records may be incomplete, inaccurate, or lacking in data needed for research analysis. When analysing secondary data, prior to undertaking the study, the researcher must establish the existence and authenticity of records relevant to the research. Access to relevant records must be negotiated, and sampling issues considered to overcome sampling bias (see Chapter 8).

Consideration must also be given to the analysis of information that was collected within one context that is to be used by the researcher in another context to address a research question. It is possible that analysis by the researcher will ignore the context in which the data were originally collected and inappropriate judgements may be made.

The increased need to record information in health care offers the researcher a wealth of information for consideration. The potential gains from such analysis have been recognised by many researchers and are likely to be considered by many more in the future, despite the potential difficulties, which arise from using and analysing secondary data.

TRIANGULATION OF DATA COLLECTION

Researchers often employ more than one methodological approach, using multiple methods to collect data. The term 'triangulation of methods' is used to imply that three or more research methods have been used in one study, often involving both quantitative and qualitative data collection methods (Moule and Goodman, 2014). For example, data collection might include using a survey with closed and open questions to ascertain client use of a new service, followed by individual interviews or focus groups with a range of stakeholders. Saurman et al. (2011) used mixed methods to evaluate a nursing intervention. They triangulated the research design to review a new mental health emergency care service delivered to remote areas. The design located a researcher with the service delivery team to gain an understanding of the ways the team worked; data on each telephone call taken from service users was collected; staff interviews were conducted; and the service users were asked to rate their experience of the service using a video assessment.

KEY POINTS

- Research information can be collected in many ways.
- The research approach taken will influence the choice of data collection instruments.
- Reliability and validity are important qualities of any data collection instrument.
- Establishing trustworthiness should be considered in qualitative research.
- Methods of analysis will need consideration prior to data collection.

FURTHER READING

Bell, J. (2010). *Doing your research project: A guide for first-time researchers in education, health and social science* (5th edn). Buckingham: Open University Press.

Bowling, A. (2009). *Measuring health: A review of quality of life measurement scales* (3rd edn). Buckingham: Open University Press.

Brace, I. (2013). *Questionnaire design: How to plan, structure and write survey material for effective market research* (3rd edn) London: Kogan Page Ltd.

Burns, N. and Grove, S. (2013). *The practice of nursing research: Appraisal, synthesis and generation of evidence* (7th edn). St Louis, MO: Saunders Elsevier.

McDowell, I. (2006). *Measuring health: A guide to rating scales and questionnaires* (3rd edn). Oxford: Oxford University Press.

Moule, P. and Goodman, M. (2014). *Nursing research: An introduction* (2nd edn) London: Sage.

Nurse Researcher (1998). *Healthcare assessment tools.* 5 (3), Spring.

Parahoo, K. (2014). *Nursing research: Principles, process and issues* (3rd edn). Basingstoke: Palgrave Macmillan.

Polit, D. and Beck, C. (2010). *Essentials of nursing research: Methods, appraisal and utilization* (7th edn). Philadelphia, PA: Lippincott Williams and Wilkins.

WEBSITES

UK Medicines information on questionnaire design: www.ukmi.nhs.uk/research/resSkillsqdesign.asp

10   MAKING SENSE OF DATA ANALYSIS

LEARNING OUTCOMES

On completion of this chapter the reader should be able to:

- understand the difference between descriptive and inferential statistics
- identify the significance of quantitative results
- appreciate the steps required to complete qualitative data analysis.

KEY CONCEPTS

- standard deviation
- levels of measurement
- parametric
- grounded theory
- measures of central tendency
- constant comparison
- non-parametric
- thematic analysis
- normal distribution

INTRODUCTION

Many professionals and students in health and social care find the results and analysis section of a research article difficult to understand. This chapter is aimed at demystifying some of the terminology used in those sections and helping those who read and interpret the findings of published research.

The type of analysis the researcher can apply to the data varies according to the approach taken, and nature of data collected. **Quantitative data analysis** is discussed in the first part of the chapter and emphasis placed on the interpretation of results. In the discussion on **qualitative data analysis** the core methods used by researchers from the various qualitative approaches will be identified and examples from current health and social care research used to illustrate points made.

DATA ANALYSIS USED IN QUANTITATIVE RESEARCH STUDIES

DESCRIPTIVE STATISTICS

When a researcher plans their research design they must have some idea of the type of **data analysis** that will match their approach to the study and the data collecting methods employed. In the first part of the data analysis section of a research article, the researcher usually makes an attempt to describe their results and put them in the context of all the responses obtained.

When asked to describe the age of a group of people, one way of doing this is to give an 'average' age of the group. This is something used in many contexts of our everyday life. Averages of different kinds are used in research articles to describe a set of responses. The type of average used depends on the type of data the researcher is working with.

Below are two questions from a questionnaire which asked students how they had travelled to university that morning, and also the distance they had travelled.

1. Please tick the box which identifies how you travelled to college this morning

Car	☐	Bus	☐	Motorcycle	☐
Train	☐	Bicycle	☐	Walk	☐
Other	☐				

2. Please identify to the nearest kilometre the distance you travelled to university this morning

These two questions will produce quite different types of data, and because of that will need different kinds of averages. In question 1, the researcher will need to add up all the respondents who ticked each of the boxes and could end up with a list such as this:

Car	64	Bus	11	Motorcycle	5
Train	0	Bicycle	7	Walk	8
Other	0				

To tell us something about the way this group of students travelled to university the researcher will have to identify the means of transport used by most students. In this case that will be car, with 64 – the most common by a long way. In statistical terms this type of data is called 'nominal' as it is collected in named categories (for example, car, train), and the researcher counts the frequency found in each category. The category that occurs most frequently is called the **mode**. If two categories have the same frequency the data is called bi-modal, and with more than two categories the term multi-modal is used.

In question 2, the respondents are asked to provide the distance they travelled to university. This is potentially an accurate measurement in which the scale used (kilometres) is recognised internationally. If one student travelled two kilometres it would be acknowledged that a student who travelled four kilometres had travelled twice as far. To tell us about the distances travelled to university by the students the researcher could calculate the average as we use it in our everyday lives; that is, add all the distances and divide that sum by the number of students. In statistical terms this type of data is called 'ratio', and the average referred to as the **mean**.

In between these two categories of data are two more. 'Ordinal' data are measurements which can be put into a rank order but are not measured on an accurate scale. This means that the researcher could put the data in order from lowest to highest or smallest to largest but that is all. A good example of this type of data is the scale used in the assessment of patients' pain. The score on a Visual Analogue Scale (see Chapter 9) used to measure a patient's pain is an example of 'ordinal' data. If one patient marked six on such a scale it could not be said that they have exactly twice the pain of a patient who marked three. However, it might be gauged that they were in more pain at the time.

Due to the inaccuracy of the measurement, a mean should not be used as an average in this type of measurement. Instead, to obtain a way of describing 'ordinal' data, all the measurements are put into a rank order, from lowest to highest or smallest to largest, and the middle measurement of the rank is identified as the **median**. So, for example, to describe the risk of re-offending of a group of young offenders the researcher would put the risk assessment scores of each young offender in a rank order, from lowest to highest, and find the score exactly in the centre. This would give some indication of the risk of re-offending by a group of young offenders.

The final category of data that may be used is 'interval' data. This is similar to 'ratio' data but a scale is used in which there is no absolute zero and therefore no fixed point. The example usually given in statistical texts is that of the Fahrenheit scale for measuring temperature. However, as this data is measured on a recognised scale the mean is the average used. Usually in health and social care research 'interval' and 'ratio' data are treated together.

These different types of data are called levels of measurement and are regarded as a hierarchy. Statisticians refer to the averages which have been described as measures of central tendency. A summary of the levels of measurement and measures of central tendency can be seen in Table 10.1.

Table 10.1 *Summary of levels of measurement and measures of central tendency (MCT)*

Date	Characteristics	MCT
Nominal	frequency of categories	mode
Ordinal	no scale but can be ranked	median
Interval	measured on a scale but no zero	mean
Ratio	most accurate, measured on scale with absolute zero	mean

When using 'interval' or 'ratio' data, researchers can go further in their ability to describe the data recorded from their sample. They can show if their sample had very similar scores, or if their scores covered a wide range. To do this the data must be put in a format where not only is the mean identified, but the number of respondents who achieved each score is also identified. Statisticians have found that if they take any measurement from a random sample of subjects there will always be a few at the extremes of a measurement scale but most will be clustered around the mean. This is most easily shown in a diagram. Figure 10.1 shows a normal distribution curve; that is, a pattern of measurements, shaped like a bell, in which the horizontal axis is the scale of measurements and the vertical axis is the frequency of each of the measurements.

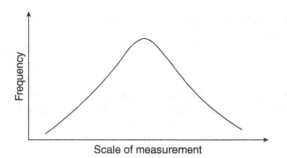

Figure 10.1   *Normal distribution curve*

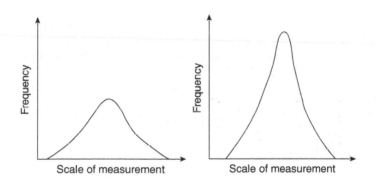

Figure 10.2   *Different distribution curves*

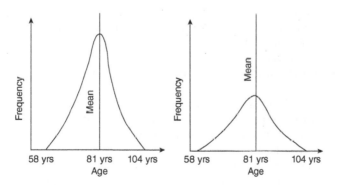

Figure 10.3   *Bell-shaped curve – patient/age distribution on elderly care ward*

This bell shape can vary between being short and fat, and tall and thin (see Figure 10.2).

The shape of the bell can tell us quite a lot about a set of results and therefore about a **sample**. To illustrate this look at Figure 10.3.

The bell on the left shows the range of ages of patients admitted to a stroke rehabilitation unit the first year after it had opened. It can be seen that ages range from 58 years (the youngest) to 104 years (the oldest) and that the mean age was 81 years.

The bell on the right shows the range of ages of patients admitted to the same unit five years later. The range of ages remains much the same and so does the mean and yet the shape of the bell is very different. The tall thin bell on the left shows that the ages of a majority of patients were very close to the mean, with very few at the extremes of the age span. However, the bell on the right shows that there were many more patients at the extremes, with far fewer patients clustered around the mean age of 81 years. When comparing these two distribution curves the researcher might begin to think of reasons why these results have been gained and the effect of these changes on the workload of the staff. Reasons for the change might include, for example, different admissions policies or the presence of other faculties in the community. The effect on the staff might include the need for a flexible approach to the use of a multidisciplinary team.

When reading research articles the mean of a set of results might be given along with another figure called the **standard deviation** (sd). The standard deviation refers to the spread of the results away from the mean. In other words, it is a numerical value given to the shape of the bell curve referred to above. The value of the standard deviation is determined by calculating the difference between each of the scores and the mean, and then finding an average difference.

As standard deviation is calculated on the more rigorous measurements of interval and ratio data, various assumptions can be made from the use of a standard deviation and the bell-shaped curve. Figure 10.4 shows a normal distribution curve with the standard deviation marked in. On each side of the mean there is one standard deviation marked: on the left it is minus one standard deviation and on the right, plus one standard deviation. This allows the researcher to predict, from the sample, the number of

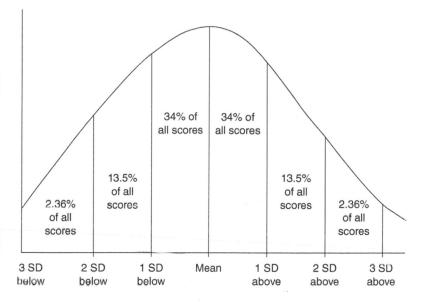

3 SD below   2 SD below   1 SD below   Mean   1 SD above   2 SD above   3 SD above

Figure 10.4   *Bell-shaped curve and standard deviation*

the population who will 'fall between' −1 and +1 and −2 and +2 standard deviations.

Sometimes the standard deviation is used to see if two groups are comparable and can be used in further statistical testing. It must be remembered that the standard deviations always read in conjunction with the mean.

It can be seen from Figure 10.4 that 68% of all cases will fall between −1 and +1 and 95% of the population between −2 and +2 standard deviations.

Another way researchers describe their results is with the aid of pictorial representation. Pie charts such as Figure 10.5 are used in nominal data to show the proportion of each category to the whole set of results.

Each slice of the pie represents one category. Sometimes the sections are simply drawn, but other times researchers will actually pull a slice of the pie out to make a particular point. A pie chart is an effective yet simple pictorial representation of a set of results which demonstrates how each segment is a proportion of a whole.

Another common representation used to describe a set of results is a bar chart. Bar charts are often used to compare differences between groups or changes in groups.

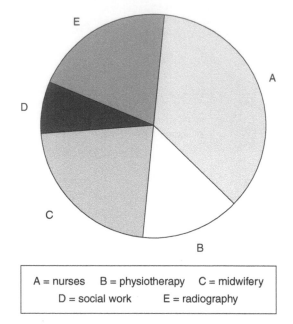

Figure 10.5   *Pie chart showing groups of students*

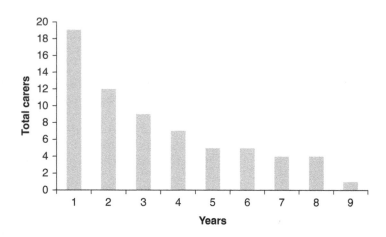

Figure 10.6   *Bar chart showing the number of years spent in a caring role*

When looking at both pie and bar charts, extremes of measurement should be noted, and the questioning process of why these results have occurred should be starting.

Figure 10.6 shows a bar chart used to describe the number of years spent caring by a population of 66 people.

Having described a set of results many researchers attempt to put some meaning into them. When reading a research article, this part of the data analysis usually follows the **descriptive statistics** and uses **inferential statistics**, or statistics which infer some meaning.

PRACTICE EXAMPLE

Moule et al. (2010) used a mixed methods approach to look at how e-learning technologies are being used in higher education environments to prepare health sciences students. Quantitative data collected was analysed using descriptive statistics, discussed here. A discussion of the analysis of the qualitative data is presented later in the chapter.

The research included two phases of data collection and analysis. The first phase included a survey of higher education institutions conducted by post. From the 93 institutions included in the initial total sample, 25 replies were received. One of the questions asked on the survey related to the use of e-learning applications. The replies to this were at a 'nominal' level. The data were coded and entered into a Statistical Package for Social Sciences (SPSS version 13) that was used for analysis. Descriptive statistics were calculated, including frequency counts and percentages. The following results show the highest and lowest reported use of e-learning:

Uses of e-learning	Number	Percent
Access to course materials	25	100%
Online student presentations	7	28%

The results are presented to show the number of institutions recording use of e-learning and the percentage of the total number of institutions this relates to. Twenty-five institutions, the total sample, use e-learning to allow student access to course materials, giving a percentage of 100. However, online student presentations are used by only seven of the twenty-five institutions, a percentage of 28. These are presented as a table, though the data could have been shown as a bar chart.

INFERENTIAL STATISTICS

In quantitative studies the researcher frequently looks for a relationship between two or more variables, or a difference between two or more groups.

Tests of a relationship (in statistical terms referred to as a correlation) are chosen according to the level of measurement of the data. The two most common correlation tests are Spearman's Rank Correlation used for ordinal data and Pearson Product Moment used on interval or ratio data. The symbols used to denote these two tests are R_s for Spearman's and r for Pearson. Regardless of the actual test used, a coefficient or figure will be calculated which shows if there is a relationship between the variables, and, if so, how strong that relationship is. A positive correlation indicates that as the measurement of one variable has increased, so has the measurement on the other variable.

A **correlation coefficient** between +0.6 and +0.9 shows a strong positive relationship. The closer the figure is to +1 the stronger the relationship. Similarly a correlation coefficient between –0.6 and –0.9 shows a strongly negative relationship. This indicates that as one measurement has increased the other has decreased. A correlation coefficient either side of 0 suggests that there is either a very loose relationship or no relationship between the variables. In their study investigating possible differences between the parents' encounter with their stillborn child, Saflund and Wredling (2006) found an association between the time the father spent with the child and the child's birth weight. The higher the weight the more time the father spent with the child (r = 0.53).

Sometimes a correlation coefficient is obtained to demonstrate **reliability** between two researchers who are working together. Comparisons of reliability between researchers/ raters are one way in which a researcher can demonstrate the robust nature of the measurements in a quantitative study. Two researchers will independently take measurements of the same **variable** and compare their results. It is expected that the correlation will be over r = 0.80.

There are many statistical tests of difference used by researchers in their attempt to demonstrate significant findings in their results. As in the measurement of central tendency and the correlation tests, the choice of tests that can be used depends on the level of measurement of the data. Tests that can be used on nominal and ordinal data are referred to as non-parametric, and are less powerful than those used on interval and ratio data, which are called **parametric tests**. Parametric tests usually need data which have a normal distribution, with samples having similarly shaped bell curves. The most common statistical test used on nominal data is chi squared (χ^2). **Non-parametric tests**, which can be used on ordinal data and look at the difference in the ranking of a data set, include the Mann Whitney U test and the Wilcoxon test. Parametric tests which are frequently seen in research literature include the t-test and ANOVA (Analysis of Variance). A further consideration the researcher has when deciding which test to use lies in the number of groups included in the study.

To be able to interpret quantitative research data it is not necessary to have an in-depth knowledge of these tests although it is necessary to understand why the tests are performed, and how the results can be interpreted. All the tests (both parametric and non-parametric) produce a number – an index, usually with an initial before it such as U or t. These initials simply identify the statistical test which was used. Most commonly the data are entered into a statistical computer package (often SPSS). The result produced by the computer looks as follows:

$p < 0.05$, $p < 0.01$, $p < 0.001$

The p stands for **probability** and it gives the researcher an insight into how significant their results are, and what the probability is that the results occurred by chance. Users of research also need to know how powerful research results are; they are rarely interested in results which could have happened by chance, or were a 'one off'. The three probability values listed are sometimes referred to as critical values, as they are the levels of significance most frequently quoted in health and social care research:

- $p < 0.05$ – is the least powerful result usually accepted as significant in health and social care research. It means five times out of a hundred these results could have occurred by chance.
- $p < 0.01$ – is a more acceptable level and refers to a one in a hundred likelihood of the result occurring by chance.
- $p < 0.001$ – is a highly significant result and the odds of these results occurring by chance has dropped to one in a thousand.

When the result is followed by ns it means that the result is non-significant. In a study by Giles and Moule (2004) nurses' attitudes to, and experiences of, 'do not attempt resuscitation' (DNAR) policy were compared with five variables (age, grade, years of nursing, area and length of experience on current ward).

Although the comparison between the variables and nurses' attitudes to DNAR decision-making was non-significant (ns), when the researchers compared the nurses' experiences of DNAR decision-making there was a significant difference found when compared to area of practice ($p < 0.01$). Nurses working in acute and general medical wards had better experiences of DNAR decision-making than colleagues did in general surgical, neurosurgical and orthopaedics/trauma.

The more research is read, including these statistical results, the more familiar the terminology will become. This part of the chapter has attempted to introduce some of the issues in quantitative data analysis in a way to help health and social care workers of all levels begin to feel more confident in reading statistical results. For a useful text on statistics see Scott and Mazhindu (2014).

PRACTICE EXAMPLE

Saflund and Wredling (2006) used a range of inferential statistical tests in the analysis of data looking at differences within couples' experiences of their hospital care three months after experiencing a stillbirth. In total 22 couples were involved in the research across Stockholm. Data were collected using two questionnaires. The tests used included a χ-square, Wilcoxon's signed rank test, Student's paired t-test and Spearman's Rank Correlation, all to look at differences between the couples' experiences. The χ-square test was performed to look for differences between the parents' rankings of the degree of support given. This type of test is used for comparing groups when 'nominal' data has been collected. The Wilcoxon's signed rank test was used to analyse different scores given by the mothers and fathers to multiple-choice questions. This test can be used to compare 'ordinal' level data. The Student's paired t-test was used to look at differences in mean scores achieved for certain scales in the questionnaire. The t-test is used to compare the mean from 'interval' or 'ratio' data. The Spearman's Rank Correlation coefficient looked at different factors measured in other scales and, as mentioned earlier, identified an association between how long the father held the child and the child's birth weight. The analysis was completed using an online statistical package and the results achieving a probability level of ≤ 0.05 were accepted as statistically significant. Gilchrist and Wright (2014) offer a fuller explanation of these tests and how their use links to the original study hypotheses.

DATA ANALYSIS USED IN QUALITATIVE RESEARCH STUDIES

In Chapter 6 it was identified that there are several qualitative approaches to research including phenomenology, **ethnography** and **grounded theory**. In Chapter 9 the various research data collecting methods used in these types of research were discussed. However the data were collected, or whatever the exact approach used, eventually the researcher will work on the written word. Following data collection, the researcher will need to transcribe taped interview recordings, and complete observation field notes. The data from open questions on a **questionnaire** will be ready to work on.

The first task of the researcher is to try to put the data into some order. This is usually done by reading and re-reading the data, and identifying some preliminary categories which emerge. While selecting these categories there is a sense that the researcher needs to both tell a story, and paint a full picture of the topic under investigation. To do that the researcher must be careful in their choice of categories. At the preliminary stages of qualitative data analysis, a colleague may be asked to read a sample of the data and identify categories. There will then be some comparison of themes and an agreement sought (see Moule and Goodman, 2014 for a fuller explanation).

Once the categories have been identified the data are scrutinised, and a coding scheme devised which incorporates all the categories found in the data. Robinson et al. (2005) undertook an investigation into couples' psychological reactions to a diagnosis of dementia of one partner. From the analysis of the data the following themes arose: (a) making sense and adjusting to loss, (b) everything's changed, we have to go from there, (c) not quite the same person. The actual coding might be completed in various ways. Some researchers mark the transcribed data with the codes. The data can be uploaded into the computer to allow basic searches for the coded categories and the retrieval of the coded segments. Computer-assisted qualitative data analysis software (CAQDAS) can help support researchers in the analysis of large amounts of qualitative data. Four of the more common computer packages available for this are ETHNOGRAPH, NUD*IST, ATLAS Ti and NVivo. Supportive information on the use of CAQDAS is available on the Economic and Social Research Council website, (www.surrey.ac.uk/sociology/research/researchcentres/caqdas). Additionally, there are texts on the use of specific packages, such as that of Bazeley and Jackson (2013), who outline the use of NVivo.

Once the data have been coded the next step is to look for common themes. These might be closely allied to the categories, or fall across the categories. Polit and Beck (2014) suggest that not only should themes be sought, but also patterns to the themes. Once these patterns have been identified the researcher might then be able to identify those themes that lie outside the patterns.

PRACTICE EXAMPLE

In phase two of the study by Moule et al. (2010) looking at the use of e-learning by higher education institutions individual interviews were conducted with 35 staff members. The interviews were recorded and transcribed verbatim. The researchers independently analysed the transcripts to identify key themes. The process of thematic analysis is described by Miles and Huberman (1994) and involved the researchers reading data to identify key words and start the process of coding. The coded transcripts were reviewed by the other team members, who agreed areas of consistency across the suggested codes. These were the themes and subcategories. The researchers were unable to use 'member checking' (asking the participants to verify the interpretations of the data) to verify the analysis. Given the amount of data collected the team could have used computer-assisted qualitative data analysis software to support online data analysis. There were two identified themes, each with sub-themes. One of the themes was 'enablers of use'. This theme represented what the participants had said helped them in trying to use e-learning to support teaching and learning. Some of the sub-themes were the institutional strategies that enabled the use of e-learning and staff champions whose support was vital in e-learning development and use.

Sometimes the analysis may be completed using the constant comparative method. In this method, themes are identified early in the examination of the data, and then the rest of the data is scrutinised looking for the themes and constantly comparing the data with the themes. Further examples of constant comparison are found in the discussion of grounded theory (Strauss and Corbin, 1997).

In his discussion on the analysis of ethnographic data, Fielding (2008) identifies that the researcher must be aware that not all data are equally important, and that some confidence must be shown in the selection of the data. Fielding continues to discuss the properties of qualitative analysis, and the need for systematically gathered data to reflect the phenomenon (Fielding, 2008). On the other hand, poor analysis that does not reflect the phenomenon is descriptive and lacking in any direction.

Unlike quantitative data analysis in which there is a need to generalise the results from a sample of the research population, qualitative data analysis does not demand **generalisability**. Rather, there is a quest to gain deeper understanding of the phenomenon under scrutiny.

Qualitative researchers attempt to increase the body of knowledge about certain phenomena. In some cases this involves examining data and identifying themes; however, other researchers plan to take their research further and actually develop theories from their data. Grounded theory, originated by Glaser and Strauss (1967), is frequently found in qualitative research. In these studies the constant comparison of themes begins soon after the first data are collected. Rather than collect the data in one stage, and then move on to the analysis as another stage, grounded theorists examine the early data straight away, and then devise categories generated by the data to focus the rest of their data collection. As more data are collected, it is hoped they will reveal more about the categories, or cast doubt on the wisdom of their selection as categories. This part of the process is called theoretical sampling, and continues until the data fail to produce any new categories or information. To help validate the emerging theory, the categories may then be applied to a different, but similar setting, to see if they stand up to testing. This is referred to as comparative sampling, and allows the data to be utilised as a body of information constantly being updated and elaborated.

PRACTICE EXAMPLE

Langfield and James (2009) used a constant comparison method to code semi-structured interview data. The research explored the ownership of fish as pets, collecting data from nine participants. The nine interviews were transcribed verbatim and both researchers coded one transcript independently. They read through the transcript identifying key points being made. They then discussed the coding and developed

(Continued)

(Continued)

an initial list of codes. The researchers kept a reflective diary and used this to inform the coding process. Information from the rest of the interviews was constantly compared through the coding process and final themes were developed from the codes. The researchers read each interview transcript, identified the codes from the data and compared them with the original coding list. Examples of the themes and codes developed included:

Theme: caring for a pet fish. *Codes:* caring, attachment, owner happiness.

Theme: reasons for owning a fish. *Codes:* appeal, fish in childhood, other pets unsuitable, gift.

Their analysis was checked by the participants and some modification of the themes occurred to reflect the feedback. This meant that the participants were acting to check and verify the final themes and codes.

CONTENT ANALYSIS

This system of analysis is almost like a bridge between qualitative and quantitative analysis, as there is some measurement involved. It is often used to analyse media coverage of a subject, although it can be used with any form of communication (for example, health promotion leaflets). When proceeding with this form of analysis, the researcher will first decide on the area of interest and then decide on the unit of analysis. This unit could be a word or centimetre of newsprint, or minutes of television coverage. It could be centimetres of newsprint devoted to headlines, compared to centimetres of newsprint devoted to the editorial. The other measurement employed might be the frequency with which a category appears within each unit of analysis. Some researchers will decide on a list of topics they want to examine, and simply sift through the data, making a note of whether or not the topic was included. **Content analysis** might be used to look at the information given to teenagers through the medium of 'teenage magazines'. The researcher would have first decided on a topic in which they were interested, for example, advice on contraception. A search of the available magazines would then be commenced, probably looking at a specific range of magazines over a specific length of time. Prior to searching the magazines the researcher would have decided on the themes they were looking for such as:

- the use of condoms
- clinics available for young people for advice
- need for safe sex and not just contraception;

or, the researcher might be interested in the mode in which any messages were conveyed, for example:

- whether the characters in the stories discuss sex or contraceptives
- whether there were editorials around the issue of contraception
- the context in which contraception was mentioned in the magazine.

Although not widely used as a means of analysis, content analysis is used in health education and promotion research, and offers a link between research and a means of communication.

It is also used in forms of **historical research**, when the data are in the form of old documents including letters and reports.

KEY POINTS

- Descriptive statistics describe results.
- Inferential statistics attempt to infer meaning from results.
- Different types of written questions produce different levels of measurement.
- The level of measurement of data dictates the measurement of central tendency and the statistical tests that can be used.
- Qualitative data analysis uses narrative to identify themes.
- In grounded theory the data collection and analysis are performed at the same time.

FURTHER READING

Bazeley, P. and Jackson, K. (2013). *Qualitative data analysis with NVivo* (2nd edn). London: Sage.

Bryman, A. and Cramer, D. (2011). *Quantitative data analysis with IBM SPSS 17, 18 & 19: A guide for social scientists*. London: Routledge.

Grbich, C. (2013). *Qualitative data analysis: An introduction* (2nd edn). London: Sage.
Miles, M. and Huberman, M. (1994). *Qualitative data analysis: An expanded resource book* (2nd edn). Thousand Oaks: Sage.
Scott, I. and Mazhindu, D. (2014). *Statistics for healthcare professionals: An introduction* (2nd edn). London: Sage.

WEBSITES

Economic and Social Research Council: www.surrey.ac.uk/sociology/research/researchcentres/caqdas
University of the West of England Data Analysis site: http://learntech.uwe.ac.uk/da/qualitativeanalysis3.aspx

11 CRITICAL APPRAISAL OF HEALTH AND SOCIAL CARE RESEARCH

LEARNING OUTCOMES

On completion of this chapter the reader should be able to:

- appreciate the need to critically appraise research and evidence
- identify the strengths and weaknesses of qualitative and quantitative research
- critically appraise a research journal article.

KEY CONCEPTS

- critical appraisal
- critiquing framework

INTRODUCTION

Individuals working in a health and social care setting need to be able to critically appraise research for many different reasons. In Chapter 1 the term 'research literate' was used as a basis for discussion. This discussion centred on the need to be able to appreciate the skills and knowledge required to understand and use research to provide a high-quality service. A result of having these skills and knowledge is the ability to be able to read and critically appraise the many research articles in journals.

Evaluative and critical skills are used in our everyday life. Every time a decision is made in the supermarket regarding the brand of toothpaste or shampoo we buy, we are influenced by sources, such as marketing, the media, our experiences, family tradition, the cost, and so on. So these skills are not new but they do need to be developed to be applied to the world of research.

Before critically appraising research it is important to recognise that this does not necessarily mean being negative. Critical appraisal, sometimes referred to as critiquing, is more about looking for strengths and weaknesses in a study and making a balanced judgment about what has been presented in the publication. Moule and Goodman (2014) suggest that research studies are not perfect and that all should be critically appraised. Being critical involves making informed judgments about the merit of a piece of research, appraising the good and bad points of research. The process should be objective and balanced and consider the significance of the research to the field.

Developing critical appraisal skills has become crucial to all professionals and students regardless of their working background. Many courses ask for a research critique or demonstration of critical appraisal skills within their assessment schemes. Some institutions of higher education include a **literature review** in their dissertation assessment which will require critically appraising many pieces of research in trying to answer a **research question**. Acquiring the skills needed to critically appraise published research depends on practice and thoughtful reading of research articles and reports. At first the language can appear alien, and sometimes the results appear to be written in a format requiring high levels of statistical knowledge to interpret. This may leave the reader feeling bewildered.

A worthwhile introduction to reading research and developing critical appraisal skills is to read several research articles which all address the same (or similar) topic. This topic should be one in which the reader is particularly interested either for an assignment or because the articles relate to a specific subject. It is surprising how an interest in a specific subject helps overcome some of the immediate challenges of reading research. The other point to recognise is that not all parts of the research paper need be understood in the first couple of readings. However, gradually, as knowledge is increased, more and more will be understood. One approach is described by Maslin-Prothero (2010) that suggests there are three levels of reading: scanning, in-depth reading and inferring. An initial skim read to decide on the section of the paper to concentrate on, is followed by in-depth reading of these sections, inferring by thinking about context and questioning the material. Appendix 2 includes the stages of critical appraisal.

In the final stages of reading a research article various questions can be asked at each stage of the research process. This helps identify both strengths and weaknesses of the study; it also breaks down the task into 'manageable chunks'. The rest of this chapter looks at various parts of the research process and identifies areas that the reader could question. A critical appraisal framework is found in Appendix 3. More detailed frameworks can be found in Moule and Goodman (2014) and on the website: www.casp-uk.net.

SETTING THE RESEARCH SCENE

In the first part of the article the author should identify the purpose of the study and why the research needs to be completed. This might be because a problem was identified or the researcher had a question they wanted to answer. Whatever the reason, all research should contribute to knowledge, either by identifying more questions to ask or by adding findings to the current body of knowledge. There needs to be some reassurance from the research that the study will fulfil this requirement and that the researcher is appropriately prepared to be conducting the study. There should be a clear purpose for the research, with a researchable problem.

Unless the researcher is using **grounded theory** and is purposely not looking at the related literature until later in the study, the literature review should provide a background to the study. In the literature review there should be a comparing and contrasting of the literature, and a critique of it rather than simply a description. The strengths and weaknesses of previous studies should be identified and the dates of the studies should be noted. Although the literature review should include any seminal work on the topic, regardless of its age, there should be an attempt to embrace the most recent work as well.

Developing from the background and literature review, the researcher should establish a focus for the study. In a quantitative study this should be a defined focus often in the form of a **hypothesis** but it might also be a question or an aim (see Chapter 7). If there is a hypothesis it should be seen to emerge from the literature and it must be relevant to the topic being studied. The wording of the hypothesis should be clear and at least two variables identified. It should also be obvious whether the researcher is looking for a relationship between two or more variables or for differences between groups. When appraising a quantitative report where a null hypothesis is tested, the reader should check to see whether a null hypothesis has been used and if the statistical analysis includes a two-tailed test of significance.

In qualitative studies there should be a focus for the study in the form of aims, questions or objectives. These can be scrutinised for their relevance to the research approach and the literature review. In both qualitative and quantitative studies the hypothesis, aims or objectives should be examined to see if they link the previous work completed in this topic area with the research about to be undertaken. By keeping this as a central focus when appraising a study the reader can often discover inconsistencies either with the literature and the approach or with the literature and the design. In order to do this the reader must be familiar with the purpose of research aims, hypotheses and questions.

PRACTICE EXAMPLE

Bobillier Chaumon et al. (2014) considered whether information and communication technology (ICT) could improve the quality of life of elderly adults living in residential home care units. The introduction to the article presents literature that supports the issues, which include the desire and benefits of remaining in one's own home, but the need for residential living by those with dependency issues. The possibilities that ICT might offer to support the elderly living in institutions is proposed and research supporting the impact on quality of life is presented. It is also made clear that there is limited research assessing the psycho-social impacts of ICT on elderly adults living in residential units. The paper then presents three hypotheses supported by the literature presented. These suggest that positive relationships are expected from the implementation and use of technologies in terms of: (1) self-esteem; (2) social integration; and (3) social practices.

When applying the critical appraisal framework (see Appendix 3) the purpose of the study is included in the introduction. Existing knowledge is presented and the rationale for the study is articulated. The three research hypotheses are developed directly from the problem and propose that there will be positive impacts from the implementation of ICT on self-esteem, social integration and social practices such as being more engaged in organised activities. The literature search includes a range of literature, pertinent to the topic area. The review includes up-to-date publications, but also some earlier work from the late 1990s, all tending to support the need for and use of ICT.

The literature search strategy is not included, though this is often the case in a research paper. The review underpins the research hypotheses, and there is evidence to suggest that ICT can impact on the psychosocial wellbeing of the elderly.

COLLECTING THE DATA AND SAMPLE SELECTION

One of the ways the researcher can demonstrate their creativity is in the design of their study. There should be some indication of how they decided on their eventual research design – the influences and the constraints. The researcher should be able to demonstrate that the chosen design is appropriate to the study. For example, Eriksson et al. (2010) used observations to study the interplay between critically ill patients and their next of kin. An alternative might have been to interview relatives and ask them how they interacted with their relatives when visiting them in an intensive care environment. However, the researcher recognised that there might be a difference between what people say they do and how they actually behave. Therefore, interviewing respondents could be seen as an inappropriate research design in this instance, even though it would have been less time consuming and expensive.

The heart of critical appraisal lies in an analysis of the way in which data were collected to solve the research problem. Therefore, in any research critique there should be an examination of alternative strategies to the one presented. Once the design has been examined the data collection methods and the **sample** used need careful scrutiny. The appropriate size of the sample will differ depending on the research approach used. In qualitative studies a small sample is used to gain in-depth information. Even with a small sample, the researcher should justify the selection of individuals. In qualitative studies the researcher might focus on particular respondents because of a specific interest. Particularly in a grounded theory approach the researcher will look at the early data received and use that to guide where they go for subsequent data. This should be explained and rationalised in the study.

When critically appraising **quantitative research** the reader should examine the sample selection very carefully. The whole thrust of studies which attempt to test a theory using a **quantitative data collection** method is the transfer of the results from the sample to the research population. In an attempt to eradicate **bias** the researcher should strive to use a random sample in which everyone in the research population has an equal chance of being included. As most research studies have constraints on them in terms of cost, a totally randomised sample is rarely seen in health and social care research. However, the implications of how the sample was selected should be included and allowed for in any discussion of the results and attempts at generalising the results. The sample should also mimic the research population in terms of its constitution. A quick look at a research study to see how the sample and research population match up in their constituent parts will give the reader an insight into the research. A researcher can only generalise to a research population that matches the sample group. When examining how the sample was selected, it is also important to examine how the participants were recruited and how they gave **informed consent**. There may have been a difference in the participants who participated and those who declined to participate or were not selected.

The data collection method should be described as well as rationalised. There may be an example of the data collection tool in the article and this allows for an examination of the **questionnaire** or interview schedule. Any measuring tool should also be included along with a discussion on how it was tested for **reliability** and validity and how the individuals collecting the data were trained in its use. At this point in the study there might be a description of the pilot study. This should indicate any changes made to the data collection tool and identify any problems the researcher found with the research design. It can take some honesty for the research to identify such problems. If results of the pilot study are not given, the reader is left unsure of what was found and somewhat insecure concerning the data collection methods used.

When evaluating a questionnaire, there needs to be an examination of the types of questions used and their relevance to the approach taken. A qualitative approach will require the interviewer to use open questions, which allow the respondent to explain exactly how they feel/think. The closed questions and measuring scales found in quantitative studies should be examined for their ease of use, their clarity and the clarity of the instructions given for their use. All questions should give respondents an opportunity to add any other thoughts they might have on the subject. In observational studies there should be some indication of the role of the observer and whether it was covert or overt observation and whether the researcher included the effect of researcher presence on any results. The researcher should also detail how the field notes were recorded and when full notes were written up.

PRACTICE EXAMPLE

Yee Chin et al. (2014) undertook a longitudinal survey in Hong Kong, which aimed to detect levels of depression in adults and explore their management. A primary care setting was used. Community doctors were invited to join a research network set up by the study. Doctors were recruited to the network using a postal list of family physicians. Patients were recruited through each doctor's practice using random selection. Each doctor was allocated recruitment days randomly and patients were invited to take part in the study on these days if they met the selection criteria (aged over 18 years, consulting the doctor, had not previously completed the study and were able to understand either English, Cantonese or Mandarin). A coded anonymous survey was completed. This included a Patient Health Questionnaire for self-reported depression, validated for use in primary care; personal data questions adapted from previous studies; and data from the standard data collection tool used by each doctor. A sample calculation was undertaken suggesting 1,540 participants were required. Ethical approval was provided by a number of hospital ethical review boards.

When applying the critical review questions (see Appendix 3), the study had sought and received appropriate ethical review. Patient consent was not discussed in the paper, though in completing and returning the questionnaires the patients were giving implied consent. The method of recruiting the doctors, through invitation to join a network interested in depression, led to a restricted sample. A random sampling process was used to recruit the patients to the study. The sample size had been determined by a sample size calculation. In total, over 10,000 patients were recruited. This equated to a response rate of 81%, as 19% of patients approached to take part declined. The data collection tools used had been previously validated and provided a resource-effective way of capturing data to answer the research questions, from the sample.

There were some limitations of the study design. As stated earlier there was a bias in sampling towards doctors with an interest in mental health, as the sample was taken from network members who had an interest in this area. In addition, whilst a random sampling strategy

(Continued)

(Continued)

was employed, the final sample included a high proportion of patients recruited from Hong Kong island, the least populated area in the region. The screening for depression was based on self-reported measures (the completion of the questionnaire by patients), rather than a clinical diagnosis of depression, which is likely to be more accurate. It is possible that involving doctors with an interest in mental health issues could have affected the results of the study; for example, there may have been improved detection rates and treatments.

RESULTS AND DATA ANALYSIS

Possibly the one aspect that many individuals feel least able to critically appraise is the result and analysis section of a research study. The first area that needs to be examined is the relevance of the results to the research approach taken. If a qualitative approach was taken the results section should demonstrate the emergence of themes from the data. Results should not necessarily offer an explanation but may simply give the reader the findings. In such research reports the researcher should indicate how the results were authenticated. This might involve **triangulation** when two methods could be used to collect the same information, for example, in-depth **interviews** and **observations** of behaviour, or the data may be returned to participants. In the search for themes from qualitative data a colleague might be asked to identify themes from a sample of the responses to see if there is agreement or participants might be involved in validating any emerging themes. The steps that have been taken to demonstrate the **trustworthiness** of the data in a qualitative study should be clear.

If a quantitative approach was taken in which the variables were measured, the results section should give the full range of responses. The beginning of the section should also identify the response rate from any questionnaires used. A description of the results might include pictorial representation, such as pie or bar charts, tables or graphs. These can help the reader get an overview of the results. However, all sections of any diagrams need to be accurately labeled otherwise the reader is left trying to guess what is being referred to. The diagrams should also be clear and able to 'stand alone'. If they require text to explain them they are usually inadequate.

In quantitative analysis the researcher should justify the use of specific statistical tests. The reader should be able to see a clear link between the research approach, the level of measurement gained from the data collection tool and the statistical tests used. The level of significance produced by the statistical testing should also be examined to ensure it is above the 5% ($p < 0.05$) level. In health and social care research if there is a greater than 5% probability that the results occurred by chance they are usually deemed non-significant (see Chapter 10).

PRACTICE EXAMPLE

Whiting (2014) wanted to explore parents' experiences of caring for a child with complex health needs. A series of semi-structured individual interviews were completed with 33 families of children with life-limiting conditions, a disability or technology dependence. The interviews were recorded and transcribed to allow verbatim analysis. The findings are presented as key themes with sub-themes relating to each of these. The themes are supported by verbatim quotes from the participants.

The themes emerged from an analysis of the interview transcripts. The interviews had been guided by a very open question, asking what it meant to be the parent of a disabled child. The parents provided their perspectives on this and a process of analysis identified the key themes. Some papers may provide more detail than offered here on aspects such as: the framework for analysis; how this was undertaken; and whether there has been any process of verification or independent review of the analysis.

CONCLUSIONS AND DISCUSSION OF RESULTS

One of the dangers in any research report is that the researcher will attribute more meaning to the results than the analysis will support. In moving from the data analysis section to the interpretation and conclusions the reader should be able to follow a logical progression. Any generalisation made by the researcher should be examined in the light of the results section and (if it is a qualitative study) the sample used. One of the most frequently seen problems with research is that of a small sample used in a quantitative study. For example, following statistical testing and finding significant results the researcher 'ignores' the size and constitution of the sample. The researcher need not be criticised for using a small sample but can be challenged for generalising the results from the sample to the research population without acknowledging the limitations of the study.

If the research has a hypothesis, the interpretation of the results should be examined in the light of it. The hypothesis should be accepted or rejected. The data may or may not support the hypothesis. Remember nothing in research is ever proven (see Chapter 7) as there is always an element of chance in the results, or there may be an error in the data collection methods.

Health and social care research should always address any implications for practice and policy. Ultimately research is about adding to a body of knowledge and that might be about, for example, the individuals who decide to be social workers or it may be about patients' perceptions of the physiotherapy treatment they receive. There should always be an identifiable link between the research undertaken and its practical application.

KEY POINTS

- It is essential that all health and social care workers develop critical appraisal skills.
- In order to understand research papers it is necessary to read them several times.
- All readers of research should use a systematic framework to appraise research papers.

FURTHER READING

Aveyard, H. (2010). *Doing a literature review in health and social care* (2nd edn). Berkshire: Open University Press

Aveyard, H. and Sharp, P. (2013). *A beginner's guide to evidence based practice in health and social care* (2nd edn). Berkshire: Open University Press.

Cottrell, S. (2011). *Critical thinking skills: Developing effective analysis and argument.* Basingstoke: Palgrave Macmillan.

Hart, C. (1998). *Doing a literature review.* London: Sage

WEBSITES

Critical Appraisal Skills Programme (CASP): www.casp-uk.net

NICE Evidence Search: www.evidence.nhs.uk

12 DISSEMINATING AND IMPLEMENTING RESEARCH

LEARNING OUTCOMES

On completion of this chapter the reader should be able to:

- recognise and appreciate the need for the dissemination of research in the health and social care professions
- identify mechanisms for dissemination of research in health and social care
- appreciate some of the problems of research utilisation in the health and social care professions
- acknowledge the responsibilities of practitioners with regard to the implementation of research as an element of evidence-based practice.

KEY CONCEPTS

- research dissemination
- research implementation
- evidence-based practice
- research utilisation

INTRODUCTION

This book has constantly highlighted the need for practitioners to recognise the importance of using research in their daily practice. The importance of nursing research for practice has been reiterated in the recent Francis Inquiry (2013) into the standards of care delivered in one NHS hospital Trust. The final report recommended the use of National Institute for Health and Care Excellence (NICE) guidelines to inform evidence-based practice and procedures (see Chapter 1). Evidence provided through research underpins the development of NICE guidance, provides the knowledge to support best and up-to-date practice, and can help reduce cost and improve patient outcomes.

The now common terms 'research literacy' and 'research awareness' have been used to describe the skills that health and social care practitioners need to enable them to gain access to relevant literature, and to be able to read and critically appraise research and other types of evidence. In developing these skills, practitioners will be able to assess the appropriateness of utilising research-based evidence in their daily practice in order to provide the highest standards of care possible. In addition, they will be able to contribute to the identification of research problems and priorities that may need to be further investigated.

Finding out about research that is relevant to practice is dealt with partly by thorough literature searching (see Chapter 5), and appraising it for quality is dealt with in Chapter 11. This chapter deals with the final stage of the research process – **dissemination** – and explores the ways in which researchers disseminate their work, and then considers the complex issue of the research–practice gap, research application and **implementation**.

DISSEMINATION OF RESEARCH

There is widespread recognition of the need for research findings to be disseminated effectively. Researchers have a responsibility to ensure that their research findings are appropriately disseminated in different forms and at different stages to address the needs of different people. These may include fellow practitioners, academic colleagues, researchers, policy-makers, and most importantly, the participants. Disseminating findings to participants might include feedback to local groups, summaries of findings to individuals, or writing an article for a magazine that service users might read.

In some types of research, for example, **feminist research** or **action research**, the commitment to disseminate and implement is much greater as this is part of the philosophy underpinning the research design and will be an important part of the research process. Those who are most able to act on the research findings in some way are likely to be practitioners, policy-makers, and perhaps the academic community through teaching students. Researchers, therefore, need to disseminate their work in places relevant to these groups and in a format likely to be of use.

One of the most common places for the dissemination of research findings is through journals as they can normally publish research within a year or two whereas a published book will take longer. Much quicker, however, is the presentation of findings at major conferences that are usually organised for specific audiences, such as sports physiotherapists, neonatal nurses, diagnostic radiographers; or on a particular topic for a multi-professional audience, such as community rehabilitation services, child protection developments, advances in diabetes. Other means of dissemination might be through continuing professional development activity, local conferences, newsletters and web pages, feedback and audit mechanisms, or through summaries of findings.

Ethical issues might arise for the researcher wanting to publish findings that may be controversial or negative, and they will need to consider the consequences of publishing or not in terms of the ethical principles identified in Chapter 4. Researchers also have a responsibility to clearly identify the implications of their research, particularly where related to practice, and many professional journals ask that this is made explicit for the readers.

The Cochrane Collaboration, established in 1993, was set up to provide information about existing research evidence. It produces the **Cochrane Library** (www.thecochranelibrary.com), which is a main source of information to aid dissemination; it is primarily an international network of people who prepare, maintain and disseminate systematic up-to-date reviews of the effectiveness of health care. The collaboration has produced nearly 6,000 reviews so far. A sister organisation, the Campbell Collaboration (www.campbellcollaboration.org), produces reviews relevant to social interventions. Currently the Campbell Collaboration has five co-ordinating groups in social welfare: Crime and Justice, Education, International Development, Methods, Social Welfare and Knowledge Transfer and Implementation (formerly User groups). These groups have responsibility for the production of systematic reviews of scientific merit. The reviews are all provided electronically through databases and on the internet to make dissemination as easy as possible. The Centre for Reviews and Dissemination (CRD) at York (www.york.ac.uk/inst/crd), part of the National Institute for Health Research, also provides a service disseminating reviews of effectiveness to key decision-makers in the health service. It undertakes systematic reviews of the effects of health and social care interventions and service delivery and organisation. The National Institute for Health and Care Excellence (NICE) produces and disseminates evidence-based clinical guidelines for health care, and the Social Care Institute for Excellence (SCIE) (www.scie.org.uk) disseminates information about particular areas of social care. Both are extensive and free online resources with publications that can be downloaded or provided as hard copies.

THE NEED TO IMPLEMENT RESEARCH INTO PRACTICE

The implementation of research into practice is not without its challenges. Rycroft-Malone et al. (2002) highlight issues of change implementation and the use of research to improve patient care. Difficulties include a lack of research awareness amongst some staff, a reluctance to change practice and complexities of practice change. However, the drive to implement evidence-based research findings is increasing, and weight has been added to these discussions through the recent Francis Inquiry report (2013). Additionally, public awareness of health research and its potential to deliver health benefits is increasing, along with a realisation that further research is needed in particular areas, such as dementia care and cancer treatments. Professionals are therefore expected to have an awareness of research and ability to access, read, appraise and implement research as part of their practice. This book has considered how to search for and review the literature (see Chapter 5) and undertake a critical appraisal of research (see Chapter 11). This chapter considers how to disseminate and implement research in practice.

HOW TO IMPLEMENT RESEARCH FINDINGS IN PRACTICE

The implementation of new practice requires the identification of accepted evidence. However, the evidence produced from a single piece of research or other single evidence source is unlikely to be used as a basis for practice change. Evidence identified through a rigorous systematic review process (see Chapter 5) can, however, form a basis for change. A more detailed discussion of the systematic review process is offered in Moule and Goodman (2014) and by others, as suggested in the further reading list.

The recommendations arising from a systematic review, such as those produced by the Cochrane Collaboration or NICE, can be used to review current practice. The process of review will vary according to the extent of change. For example, a change that has the potential to impact many areas of an organisation, such as the NICE guidelines (2007), published by the former National Institute for Clinical Excellence on 'how to help employees stop smoking', will need addressing by the entire institution or workplace. Some practice-based changes may have relevance for a specific care team or service and will need focused discussion and change. For example, critical care teams would review the new protocol for the 'management of unstable angina' published by the former National Institute for Clinical Excellence, prior to making any practice change (NICE, 2010b). Some recommended changes may be implemented immediately, such as those to manual handling advice or resuscitation guidelines.

Nutley and Davies (2000) identify a number of strategies that have been used for changing individual and organisation practice. These include strategies aimed at individual professionals, such as opinion leaders; production of educational material; strategies aimed at organisations through reorganising skill mix; developing multidisciplinary teams; regulatory interventions; financial interventions; and patient-orientated interventions, such as involving service users and carers in decision-making. Other strategies to encourage research implementation might include joint appointments across research and practice, and practice appointments with a research component, for example, consultant nurses, or consultant physiotherapists.

The use of change theories can also support successful practice and policy guidance implementation. One approach used in the NHS is the Plan, Do Study, Act (PDSA) cycle, presented by the NHS Institute for Innovation and Improvement (www.institute.nhs.uk). The cycle can be used to trial a change and assess its impact. The cycle commences with planning the change to be tested or implemented; carrying out the test or implementing change; collecting data that measure the effect of the change and consider the learning; using the learning to develop the next change cycle or to support full implementation of the change. This approach was used in evaluating the Pacesetters programme. The programme was a partnership between the local communities, NHS and the Department of Health that aimed to deliver equality and diversity improvements and innovations that reduced health inequalities for service users and involved them in the design and delivery of services. The PDSA cycle was employed to implement a number of initiatives and evaluate and capture learning (Moule et al., 2013).

It is clear that the dissemination and implementation of research is a complex **phenomenon** and changing practice requires more than just the dissemination of findings through reports, journals, conferences and other forums. However, practitioners are a powerful group who have a responsibility to consider both the ways in which evidence can make a difference to the care of service users and carers, and how a change in practice might be made. New ways of implementing research in everyday work are now being considered, including: the ongoing development of integrated care pathways; quality improvement processes; auditing techniques; and computer support systems. Research is being conducted to identify how effective different approaches to implementation might be in changing the behaviour of health and social care professionals. A key message from all the work in this area is that single interventions do not work as well as multifaceted interventions, and that there needs to be understanding about individual decision-making and behavioural change in order to effectively get research into practice.

WAYS TO DISSEMINATE YOUR RESEARCH

The dissemination of project work, dissertations, doctoral theses and all research activity is important and should be encouraged and supported by supervisors, mentors and research funders. There are often opportunities to disseminate research findings locally. Many higher education and health care providers host research seminars and research/journal clubs, all offering an opportunity for local presentations. These events can provide an opportunity to present findings to local staff and the public. The events can be a good way to start presenting work and build up presentation skills and confidence. Further ways to present research findings include poster presentations and displays in clinical and other areas. Leaflets describing research activity provide another dissemination method.

Those who are more ambitious may want to submit an abstract to present a poster or paper at a national or international conference. If taking this route the conference call, often distributed through email, should be reviewed carefully. Most conferences have a particular focus, such as critical care or nurse education, and also invite abstract submission for particular themes, such as public engagement, simulation and technology enhanced learning. The submission should make clear which theme the abstract relates to and must meet any specific requirements, such as word length.

A range of new technologies such as a podcast or webinar can also be used to disseminate research findings. In addition, there may be scope to provide information for the public and professionals through events such as science cafés or through service user group meetings.

Authoring a journal paper can provide an opportunity to disseminate research findings to a national and international audience. There are a wide number of journals publishing health and social care research, both open access (available to the reader online without any financial or legal penalty) and subscription. Before writing a paper for publication the author should obtain a copy of the journal contributor's guidelines, generally available online. Novice writers will benefit from the support of more experienced authors, who can offer guidance on both the presentation and content of the paper. Papers are usually submitted electronically and as part of the submission process the authors will need to provide a statement to authenticate author contributions. The paper is normally subjected to editorial and peer review processes, which can take a number of weeks. Authors are notified of the outcome of the review and may be required to make minor or major changes (addressing reviewer comments); however, the paper can be accepted without change or rejected. If rejected, feedback will be provided, which can help the authors decide what actions to take next – such as re focusing the paper for submission to another journal. Further information on the dissemination of research findings can be found in Moule and Goodman (2014).

KEY POINTS

- Research findings need to be effectively disseminated by researchers.
- Implementation of research findings can be challenging and various strategies can be used to change practice.
- All health and social care practitioners have a responsibility to utilise research-based evidence in their practice.

FURTHER READING

Clifford, C. and Clarke, J. (eds) (2004). *Getting research into practice*. Edinburgh: Churchill Livingstone.

Droogan, J. and Cullum, N. (2010). Systematic reviews in nursing. In Griffiths, P. and Bridges, J. (eds), *Nursing Research Methods* (pp. 363–78). London: Sage.

Evans, D. and Pearson, A. (2010). Systematic reviews: gatekeepers of nursing knowledge. In Griffiths, P. and Bridges, J. (eds), *Nursing Research Methods* (pp. 379–90). London: Sage.

Moule, P. and Goodman, M. (2014). *Nursing research: An introduction* (2nd. edn). London: Sage.

WEBSITES

Campbell Collaboration: www.campbellcollaboration.org
Centre for Reviews and Dissemination: www.york.ac.uk/inst/crd/
Cochrane Collaboration: www.thecochranelibrary.com
National Institute for Health and Care Excellence: www.nice.org.uk
National Institute for Health Research: www.nihr.ac.uk/pages/default.aspx
NHS Institute for Innovation and Improvement: www.institute.nhs.uk
Social Care Institute for Excellence: www.scie.org.uk

APPENDIX 1 LITERATURE SEARCHING

SOURCES OF RESEARCH LITERATURE

- Systematic reviews are really important sources of research literature on a specific topic. The Cochrane Library (www.thecochraneli brary.com) is the best source of systematic reviews on health care effectiveness and the Social Care Institute of Excellence (www.scie. org.uk) produces reviews that evaluate existing research and literature about particular aspects of health care.
- Journals that contain comprehensive research articles such as: *British Journal of Learning Disabilities, British Journal of Radiology, International Journal of Therapy and Rehabilitation, Journal of Family Therapy, Health and Social Care in the Community, Physiotherapy, Research on Social Work Practice, Journal of Advanced Nursing, Intensive and Critical Care Nursing, Journal of Clinical Nursing.*
- Journals that specialise in reviewing research such as: *Cochrane Reviews* (www.cochrane.org), *Effective Health Care Bulletins* (www. york.ac.uk/inst/crd/ehcb.htm), *Evidence-based Medicine* (www.open clinical.org/ebm.htm), *Evidence-based Mental Health* (www.ebmh. bmj.com), *Evidence-based Nursing* (www.ebn.bmj.com), *Journal of Social Service Research* (www.informaworld.com/smpp/title~content =t792306968~db=all).
- Published research reports and reviews from various organisations such as: government departments, professional bodies, university departments (e.g., University of York Social Policy Research Unit, www.york.ac.uk/inst/crd/ehcb_em.htm), research units, specialist units, reports for the funders of research (e.g., National Institute for Health Research, www.nihr.ac.uk/research), charities and voluntary organisations (e.g., Joseph Rowntree Foundation Reports, www.jrf. org.uk/oublications).
- Conference papers that have been produced as a result of a national or international conference and put into a single document, journal article or are available online.
- Specialist books that report research studies on a specific subject topic. Usually the books are edited and each chapter has a different author who has undertaken research in the subject area.

- Theses and dissertations that are produced as the result of research undertaken for a degree. These are usually available at the university where the degree or doctorate was undertaken and can be borrowed for a short while or may be available online.

OTHER USEFUL INFORMATION RESOURCES

- Online databases that can be used to search for research and evidence such as: Allied and Complementary Medicine, Applied Social Services Index and Abstracts (ASSIA), British Nursing Index (BNI), Cumulative Index to Nursing and Allied Health Literature (CINAHL), Cochrane Library, Index to Theses, The Excerpta Medical Database (EMBASE), Medical Literature online (MEDLINE), National Research Register (NRR) Psychology Information (PsychINFO).

Internet resources – there are many internet sites that act as gateways to the large amount of information available. Local health and social care libraries will be able to give up-to-date information, for example:

- The King's Fund Library, which is concerned with health care and organisational management (www.kingsfund.org.uk/library).
- National Institute for Health and Care Excellence (NICE) for clinical guidelines, technology appraisals and public health guidance (www.nice.org.uk).
- Centre for Reviews and Dissemination (CRD) at York keeps a database of good-quality research reviews of the effectiveness and cost-effectiveness of health care interventions, and the management and organisation of health services. It also keeps a database of published economic evaluations of health care interventions (www.york.ac.uk/inst/crd/).

APPENDIX 2   THREE STAGES IN CRITICAL APPRAISAL

1. Complete a quick read through to decide whether the study is relevant to the topic you are investigating.
2. Read the article in-depth, identify the different parts of the study and how they relate to the whole article overall. Appraise each part of the study using a critical appraisal tool (see Appendix 3) as a guide. The tool includes a number of questions to help you appraise the strengths and weaknesses of the study.
3. Review your appraisal of each part of the study and draw these together to identify the relationships between the different parts and form conclusions about the whole study. Consider the relevance of the findings for practice.

There are a number of frameworks available to support the critical appraisal of a wide range of papers, such as Moule and Goodman (2014) and the Critical Appraisal Skills Programme (CASP): www.casp-uk.net/.

APPENDIX 3   CRITICAL APPRAISAL FRAMEWORK

THE PURPOSE OF THE STUDY

- Is the knowledge sought already available?
- Is there an important reason for the research to be undertaken?
- Are the potential outcomes of the study realistic?
- Was the researcher(s) appropriately qualified/supported to undertake the research?
- Are there any concerns about any funders of the research in relation to the process of the research described?

RESEARCH PROBLEM AND RESEARCH QUESTIONS

- Is the problem significant and researchable and have all potential ways of solving the problem been considered?
- Are all research questions and hypotheses developed directly from the problem?
- Did the research place unethical or unrealistic demands on participants?

LITERATURE SEARCH AND REVIEW

- Was there a search of a wide range of literature pertinent to the topic?
- Was there a search strategy with named databases and key search terms?
- Was the review balanced and not biased?
- Was the literature critically appraised?
- Was any conflicting evidence clearly presented?
- Did the literature review provide rationale and direction for the research?
- Is the literature review up to date?
- Were any limitations of the literature identified?

ETHICAL ISSUES

- Ethical issues should be considered at all stages of the study.
- Is there evidence of approval from the appropriate Research Ethics Committee?
- Were any governance issues dealt with appropriately?
- There should be clear evidence that privacy, dignity, anonymity and confidentiality were maintained throughout the study.
- The researcher should have identified ethical issues related to the study.
- Were any participants fully informed about the nature of the research?

SAMPLE SELECTION

- Was an appropriate sampling strategy used?
- If a random sample was selected, was it genuinely random?
- Were any biases in the sample group identified?
- Was the target population identified in a quantitative study?
- Was there a clear account of how participants were recruited and selected to take part in the study?
- Was there any coercion in recruiting participants?
- Was there clear evidence that participants gave informed consent?
- If the participants were vulnerable, has this been clearly considered in the study?
- Were all the participants accounted for throughout the study, i.e., was any attrition noted and discussed?

RESEARCH DESIGN AND DATA COLLECTION

- Was the design of the study appropriate to the research questions?
- Was an appropriate method of data collection used?
- Are the advantages and disadvantages of the method(s) discussed?
- Were the participants protected from physical and psychological harm?
- Was the issue of 'deception' dealt with appropriately in observational studies?
- Were the data gathered by appropriate people?
- Was the researcher's role and relationship with the participants fully considered?
- Were the data authenticated in qualitative studies?

RESULTS AND ANALYSIS OF FINDINGS

- Were the results and analysis linked back to the original research question?
- Were the results and analysis manipulated in order to favour particular findings?
- Was there any evidence of lost data?
- Was there evidence of a statistician's input into complex quantitative analysis?

CONCLUSIONS, RECOMMENDATIONS AND LIMITATIONS

- Were the conclusions and recommendations based on the results of the study?
- Was it clear that there was no intention to mislead or give false conclusions?
- Was the sample selected considered in relation to the recommendations?
- Did the researcher acknowledge any limitations?
- Were limitations of the findings of the study identified, as well as limitations of the study design and techniques?

GENERAL POINTS

- The researcher should acknowledge sources of support and funding.
- When critically appraising research, readers should acknowledge their own limitations and gain assistance when necessary.
- The role of service users and carers in the research should be explained.

See the companion website for more resources on critical appraisal.

GLOSSARY

Abstract	a brief summary of a piece of research which identifies the main stages of the research process.
Action research	an approach to research which attempts to bring about change as a result of reflection on practice. The researcher works alongside practitioners in order to effect change.
Anonymity	ensuring non-identification of research subjects or organisations, so that they cannot be linked with the data being collected.
Bias	an unintentional influence or effect which may occur at any stage of the research process and which distorts the findings, e.g., sample bias, interview bias.
Case study	in-depth study of an individual or organisation or event.
Cochrane Library	an electronic library of databases which include systematic reviews of the effectiveness of health care.
Common sense	knowledge that is commonly accepted.
Concept	an abstract idea which may be informed by previous experience or knowledge.
Confidentiality	ensuring data are used only for the purpose for which they are gathered and that information gathered cannot be linked to an individual.
Content analysis	the processing and interpretation of non-numerical data, e.g., examining text in great depth for recurring words or themes.
Control group	subjects that do not receive an intervention or treatment in an experiment.
Correlation coefficient	a figure calculated to demonstrate the size and direction of relationship between two variables.

Critically appraise	identifying the strengths and weaknesses of evidence by systematically considering the research processes, and making judgements about relevance and application to practice.
Data analysis	the processing, summarising and interpretation of raw data into meaningful information.
Dependent variable	the variable that is observed as the *effect* of manipulation by an independent variable.
Descriptive statistics	the use of various statistical techniques to describe numerical data, e.g., mean, standard deviation, variance.
Dissemination	ensuring the results of research are communicated to a wide audience.
Ethnography	a research approach which usually involves the researcher studying individuals or groups in their natural setting.
Evaluation research	investigating how a policy or new practice is working.
Evidence-based practice	practice that is based on current best evidence professional expertise and experience, and the patients' preference.
Experiment	a scientific research design which tests a hypothesis and whereby subjects are randomly allocated to different groups (see: control group; experimental group).
Experimental group	subjects that receive an intervention or treatment in an experiment.
External validity	the extent to which findings can be generalised to other populations or situations.
Feminist research	a particular research approach which seeks to empower women.
Gatekeeper	a term often used to describe a person or persons who are attempting to safeguard the interests of others.
Generalisability	the degree to which the researcher can transfer research findings from the studied sample to a target population.

Grounded theory	a qualitative approach to research which uses the process of inductive reasoning to develop theory from specific observations.
hawthorne effect	an effect which occurs as a result of subjects knowing they are involved in a study.
Historical research	research that aims to discover facts and understand past events.
Hypothesis	a measurable statement which sets out the expected relationship between two or more variables.
Implementation	the development of techniques to promote and support the utilisation of research.
Independent variable	in experimental research, the independent variable is the variable that is manipulated, and is thought to be the *cause* (in a cause and effect relationship).
Inferential statistics	the use of various statistical techniques either to infer meaning from the sample to the target population or to demonstrate the strength of a relationship between variables.
Informed consent	obtaining verbal or written permission from an individual to voluntarily take part in a study.
Interviews	a data collection technique that involves gathering information through verbal communication, often using a schedule, e.g., telephone interviewing, one-to-one interviews, group interviews.
Intuition	insight that is developed through experience.
Likert scale	a refined measurement scale that requires the respondent to give opinions on a series of statements.
Literature review	a section of a report, or a whole report where previous research or literature on a specific subject has been evaluated or appraised.
Literature search	systematic and thorough exploration of literature (e.g., journal articles, books, reports) on a specific subject.

Longitudinal research	a study by which the same subjects are studied at different points over a period of time.
Mean	the arithmetic average of a set of scores.
Median	the mid-point in a set of ranked scores.
Medical model	approach to health care which is derived from medical knowledge and practice.
Meta-analysis	a statistical technique which summarises results from several studies into a single estimate.
Mixed methods	using different data collection methods in addressing research questions within one study, often including qualitative and quantitative methods.
Mode	the most frequently occurring characteristic in a data set. Where two characteristics occur most frequently, the term bi-modal is used.
Non-parametric tests	a group of statistical tests used to identify differences or relationships between variables. Suitable for ordinal or nominal data.
Non-participant observation	a technique for gathering observational data where the researcher is detached from the situation being studied.
Non-probability sample	the researcher is unable to state the statistical likelihood of a member of the target population appearing in the sample. The selection of the samples was by non-random techniques.
Null hypothesis	a statement that predicts that there will be no relationship between identified variables. Sometimes known as a statistical hypothesis.
Observation	a data collection technique that involves gathering information through visual means, e.g., watching, sometimes using a schedule to record the observations.
Parametric tests	a group of sensitive and powerful statistical tests used to identify differences or relationships between variables and which are applied to interval or ratio levels of measurement.

Participant observation	a technique for gathering observational data where the researcher is part of the situation being studied.
Patient and public involvement in research	refers to involving patients and members of the public in research projects.
Phenomenon	an event studied by the researcher.
Phenomenology	a research approach which examines the lived experiences of individuals from their own perceptions.
Pilot study	a small preliminary study that allows the researcher to test the research methodology, e.g., data collection techniques.
Probability	the likelihood of research findings occurring by chance, which may be identified by a p value.
Probability sample	a sample selected randomly, allowing the researcher to state the statistical likelihood of a member of the target population appearing in the sample.
Qualitative data analysis	processing and interpretation of non-numerical data, e.g., words and text.
Qualitative data collection	gathering non-numerical data such as words and text, through various techniques, e.g., interviews and observations.
Quantitative data analysis	processing and interpretation of numerical data.
Quantitative data collection	gathering primarily numerical data through various techniques, e.g., structured questionnaires, measuring scales, physiological measurements.
Quasi-experiment	an experiment-like study which is not able to conform to all the requirements of an experiment.
Questionnaire	a data collection instrument composed of written questions that require written responses.
Randomised controlled trial	an experiment conducted in a practice environment.

Raw data	before any processing, the information that has been systematically collected by the researcher.
Reflective practice	systematically looking back and learning from past practice and experience.
Reliability	the extent to which an instrument or technique shows consistency of measurement.
Repertory grid	a technique used to elicit perceptions.
Representative sample	the degree to which a sample has the characteristics of the research population.
Research Ethics Committee	an independent group of people who meet regularly with a common aim of judging the appropriateness and scientific merit of proposed research.
Research governance	procedures for ensuring that research conducted within the health and social services is of high scientific quality, is properly managed, is in the interests of service users, has had an independent ethical review, and is appropriately monitored.
Research question	a specific question that the researcher is seeking the answer to through investigation.
Retrospective study	examining data that have been collected in the past. It is often used for the purpose of establishing a relationship between variables.
Rituals	routine and unquestioned actions.
Sample	a portion or part of a population, from which data can be collected.
Sampling	the techniques used to select a portion or part of a population.
Sampling bias	over- or under-representation of characteristics of the target population found in the sample.
Sampling error	problems resulting from the sampling technique, which lead to the generation of a biased sample.
Sampling frame	a record of all members of the population from which a sample can be selected.

Scientific knowledge	knowledge verified by systematic and rigorous enquiry.
Search strategy	the method used for searching for evidence/research to answer a particular question.
Secondary data	the extraction and use of data that have been previously collected for another purpose, e.g., hospital admission rates.
Snowball sample	approach used to access a hidden sample. The researcher needs to use networks
Snowballing	finding a few key articles, then sourcing relevant references from those articles to find others and so on until saturation.
Sources of knowledge	different types of knowledge that can be used as a basis for decision-making.
Standard deviation	a figure calculated to identify the spread of the data set around the mean.
Statistical significance	the extent to which results are 'real' rather than due to chance.
Systematic literature review	a systematic process of locating, critically appraising and synthesising literature with the aim of producing an overview.
Tacit knowledge	developed through the experience of practice over a period of time, part of 'expert opinion'.
Target population	the entire membership of the group in which the researcher is interested and from which data can be collected.
Theory	a structured collection of ideas or concepts which seeks to explain or describe phenomena.
Tradition	continued use of past actions or customs which may or may not have lost their meaning.
Trial and error	trying different ways of solving a problem until a solution is found.
Triangulation	the use of two or more research approaches, data collection methods or analysis techniques in the same study.

Trustworthiness	a term used when appraising qualitative research when describing credibility, dependability and transferability.
Validity	the extent to which an instrument or technique measures what it is intended to measure.
Variable	a characteristic that varies between individuals and can be measured or manipulated in the research, e.g., age, pain, height, gender.
Vignette	short description of a scenario, situation, case study or topic, which is used to prompt data collection.
Visual analogue scale (VAS)	a scale used to measure certain clinical symptoms, feelings and attitudes by getting participants to indicate severity of a straight line such as the level of pain experienced.

REFERENCES

Agan, D. (1987). Intuitive knowledge as a dimension of nursing. *Advanced Nursing Science*, 10 (1), 63–70.

Assil, S. and Zeidan, Z. (2013). Prevalence of depression and associated factors among elderly Sudanese: a household survey in Khartoum State. *Eastern Mediterranean Health Journal*, 19 (5), 435–40.

Argyris, L. and Schön, D. (1974). *Theory in practice*. San Francisco, CA: Jossey Bass.

Bazeley, P. and Jackson, K. (2013). *Qualitative data analysis with NVivo*. (2nd edn). London: Sage.

Beck, C. (1994). Phenomenology: its use in nursing research. *International Journal of Nursing Studies*, 31 (6), 499–510.

Bell, J. (2010). *Doing your research project: A guide for first time researchers in education, health and social science* (5th edn). Buckingham: Open University Press.

Benner, P. (1984). *From novice to expert: Excellence and power in clinical nursing practice*. Menlo Park, CA: Addison-Wesley.

Bergen, A. and While, A. (2000). A case for case studies exploring the use of the case study design in community nursing research. *Journal of Advanced Nursing*, 31 (4), 926–34.

Bobillier Chaumon M.-C., Michel, C., Bernard, F. and Croisile, B. (2014). Can ICT improve the quality of life of elderly adults living in residential home care units? From actual impacts to hidden artifacts. *Behaviour and Information Technology*, 33 (6), 574–90.

Bowling, A. (2009). *Measuring health: A review of quality of life measurement scales* (3rd edn). Buckingham: Open University Press.

Brace, I. (2013). *Questionnaire Design: How to plan, structure and write survey material for effective market research* (3rd edn). London: Kogan Page Ltd.

Bruns, R., Junior, E., Nardozza, M., Martins, W. and Moron, A. (2012). Measurement and planes assessed during second-trimester scans in Brazil: an online survey. *The Journal of Maternal-Fetal and Neonatal Medicine*, 25 (11), 2242–7.

Burnard, P. (1989). The sixth sense. *Nursing Times*, 85 (50), 52–3.

Burns, N. and Grove, S. (2007). *Study guide for understanding nursing research* (4th edn). St Louis, MO: Saunders Elsevier.

Burns, N. and Grove, S. (2013). *The practice of nursing research: Appraisal, synthesis and generation of evidence* (7th edn). St Louis, MO: Saunders Elsevier.

Cameron, L. and Murphy, J. (2006). Obtaining consent to participate in research: the issues involved in including people with a range of learning and communications disabilities. *British Journal of Learning Disabilities*, 35, 113–20.

Chan, M.-F. and Arthur, D. (2009). Nurses' attitudes towards perinatal bereavement care. *Journal of Advanced Nursing*, 65 (12), 2532–41.

Chen, Y.-M. (2010). Perceived barriers to physical activity among the older adults residing in long-term care institutions. *Journal of Clinical Nursing*, 19, 432–9.

Commission on Nursing and Midwifery (2010). *Frontline Care: report by the Prime Minister's Commission on the Future of Nursing and Midwifery in England*. London: Prime Minister's Commission on Nursing and Midwifery.

Cook, J.A. and Fonow, M. (1986). Knowledge and women's interest: issues of epistemology and methodology in feminist sociological research. *Sociological Enquiry*, Winter, 2–29.

Comeaux, T. and Steele-Moses, S. (2013). The effect of complementary music therapy on patient's postoperative state anxiety, pain control and environmental noise satisfaction. *MEDSURG Nursing*, 22 (5), 313–18.

Cunningham, R., Walton, M., Goldstein, A., Chermack, S., Shope, J., Bingham, R., Zimmerman, M. and Blow, F. (2009). Three-month follow-up of brief computerised and therapist interventions for alcohol and violence among teens. *Academic Emergency Medicine*, 16 (11), 1193–207.

Damery, S., Clifford, S. and Wilson, S. (2010). Colorectal cancer screening using the faecal occult blood test (FOBt): a survey of GP attitudes and practice in the UK. *BMC Family Practice*, 11 (20), 1–10.

Darzi, A. (2008). *High quality care for all: NHS Next Stage Review final report*. London: The Stationery Office.

Davies, H.T.O., Nutley, S.M. and Smith, P. (eds) (2000). *What Works? Evidence-based policy and practice in public services*. Bristol: The Policy Press.

Department of Health (2005). *Research governance framework for health and social care*. (2nd edn). London: DH. www.dh.gov.uk (accessed 5 May 2014).

Eriksson, T., Lindahl, B. and Bergbom, I. (2010). Visits in an intensive care unit: an observational hermeneutic study. *Intensive and Critical Care Nursing*, 26 (1), 51–7.

Farnell, S., Maxwell, L., Tan, S., Rhodes, A. and Philips, B. (2005). Temperature measurement: comparison of non-invasive methods used in adult critical care. *Journal of Critical Nursing*, 14 (5), 632–9.

Fielding, N. (2008). Ethnography. In Gilbert, N. (ed.), *Researching social life* (3rd edn) (pp. 266–84). London: Sage.

Fisher, R. (1971) *The design of experiments* (9th edn). New York: Hafner.

Francis, R. (2013). *Report of the Mid-Staffordshire NHS Trust: Public Inquiry.* London: Department of Health

Gharaibeh, H. and Mater, F.K. (2009). Young Syrian adults' knowledge, perceptions and attitudes to premarital testing. *International Nursing Review,* 56 (4), 450–5.

Gilchrist, M. and Wright, C. (2014). Quantitative data analysis (edited chapter). In Moule, P. and Goodman, M. *Nursing research: an introduction* (pp. 384–404). London: Sage.

Giles, H. and Moule, P. (2004). 'Do not attempt resuscitation' decision making: a study exploring the attitudes and experiences of nurses. *Nursing in Critical Care,* 9 (3), 115–22.

Glaser, B. and Strauss, A. (1967). *The discovery of grounded theory: Strategies for qualitative research.* Chicago, IL: Aldine.

Glicken, M. (2005). *Improving the effectiveness of the helping professions: An evidence-based approach to practice.* Thousand Oaks, CA: Sage.

Gomm, R., Hammersley, M. and Foster, P. (eds) (2000). *Case study method.* London: Sage.

Greenwood, J. (1993). Reflective practice: a critique of the work of Argyris and Schön. *Journal of Advanced Nursing,* 18 (8), 1183–7.

Guba, E. and Lincoln, Y. (1982). Epistemological and methodological bases of naturalistic enquiry. *Educational Communication and Technology,* 30 (4), 233–52.

Gunilla, C., Drew, N., Dahlberg, K. and Lutzen, K. (2002). Uncovering tacit caring knowledge. *Nursing Philosophy,* 3 (20), 144–51.

Hammersley, M. and Atkinson, P. (2007). *Ethnography: Principles in practice* (3rd edn). New York: Taylor Francis.

Hanson, E.J. and Clarke, A. (2000). The role of telematics in assisting family carers and frail older people at home. *Health and Social Care in the Community,* 8 (2), 129–37.

Haralambos, M. and Holborn, M. (2008). *Sociology, themes and perspectives* (6th edn). London: Collins.

Harding, S. (1987) *Feminism and methodology: social science issues,* cited in Webb, C. (1993). Feminist research definitions, methodology, methods and evaluation. *Journal of Advanced Nursing,* 18 (3), 416–423.

Hek, G., Langton, H. and Blunden, G. (2000). Systematically searching and reviewing literature. *Nurse Researcher,* 7 (3), 40–57.

Heneweer, H., van Woudenberg, N., van Genderen, F., Vanlees, L. and Wittink, H. (2010). Measuring psychological variables in patients with (sub) acute low back pain complaints at risk for chronicity: a validation study of the acute low back pain screening questionnaire – Dutch language version. *Spine,* 35 (4), 447–452.

Higher Education Statistics Agency (2005). cited in the UK Clinical Research Collaboration (UKCRC) (2007). *Developing the best research professionals. Qualified graduate nurses: Recommendations for preparing and supporting clinical academic nurses of the future.* London: UKCRC, p. 17.

Holloway, I. and Wheeler, S. (2002). *Qualitative research in nursing* (2nd edn). Oxford: Blackwell Science.

Involve (2012). *Involve strategy 2012–2015.* Available at: www.invo.org. uk (accessed 12 April 2014).

Janicek, M. (2006). The art of soft science: evidence-based medicine, reasoned medicine or both? *Journal of Education in Clinical Practice,* 12, 410–19.

Kelly, E. and Nisker, J. (2010). Medical students' first clinical experiences of death. *Medical Education,* 44 (4), 421–8.

Kent, P., Marks, D., Pearson, W. and Keating, S. (2005). Does clinician treatment choice improve the outcomes of manual therapy for non specific low backpain? A meta-analysis. *Journal of Manipulative and Physiological Therapeutics,* 28 (5), 312–22.

Kirby, S. (2004). A historical perspective on the contrasting experiences of nurses as research subjects and research activists. *International Journal of Nursing Practice,* 10 (6), 272–9.

Kitzinger, C. (2004). Feminist approaches. In Seale, C., Gobo, J., Gubrium, J. and Silverman, D. (eds), *Qualitative research in practice* (pp.125–40). London: Sage.

Langfield, J. and James, C. (2009). Fishy tales: experiences of the occupation of keeping fish as pets. *British Journal of Occupational Therapy,* 72 (8), 349–56.

Lincoln, Y. and Guba, E. (1985). *Naturalistic enquiry.* Newbury Park, CA: Sage.

Lincoln, Y. and Guba, E. (1986). Research evaluation and policy analysis: heuristics for disciplined enquiry. *Policy Studies Review,* 5, 546–64.

Maslin-Prothero, S. (2010). *Baillière's study skills for nurses and midwives* (4th edn). London: Baillière Tindall

McCrow, J., Beattie, E., Sullivan, K. and Fick, D. (2013). Development and review of vignettes representing older people with cognitive impairment. *Geriatric Nursing,* 34 (2), 128–37.

Melynk, B. and Fineout-Overholt, E. (2005). *Evidence-based practice in nursing and healthcare: A guide to best practice.* Philadelphia, PA: Lippincott Williams and Wilkins.

Merrell, J., Kinsella, F., Murphy, F., Philpin, S. and Ali, A. (2006). Accessibility and equity of health and social care services: exploring the views and experiences of Bangladeshi carers in South Wales, UK. *Health and Social Care in the Community,* 14 (3), 197–205.

Miles, M. and Huberman, M. (1994). *Qualitative data analysis: An expanded resource book* (2nd edn). Thousand Oaks, CA: Sage.

Mirza, I., Tareen, A., Davidson, L. and Rahman, A. (2009). Community management of intellectual disabilities in Pakistan: a mixed methods study. *Journal of Intellectual Disability Research,* 53 (6), 559–70.

Moloney, M., Aycock, D., Cotsonis, G., Myerburg, S., Farino, C. and Lentz, M. (2009). An internet-based migraine headache diary: issues in internet-based research. *Headache: The Journal of Head and Face Pain*, 49 (5), 673–86.

Moule, P. and Goodman, M. (2014). *Nursing research: An introduction* (2nd edn). London: Sage.

Moule, P. Evans, D. and Pollard, K. (2013). Using the plan-do-study-act model: pacesetters experiences. *International Journal of Healthcare Quality Assurance*, 26 (7), 593–600.

Moule, P., Ward, R. and Lockyer, L. (2010). Issues with e-learning in nursing and health education in the UK: are new technologies being embraced in the teaching and learning environments? *Journal of Research in Nursing*, 15 (4), 1–14.

National Institute for Health and Clinical Excellence (NICE) (2007). *Workplace health promotion: How to help employees stop smoking.* London: NICE.

National Institute for Health and Clinical Excellence (NICE) (2010a). *Venous thromboembolism: Reducing the risk.* London: NICE.

National Institute for Health and Clinical Excellence (NICE) (2010b). *CG94 unstable angina and NSTEMI.* London: NICE.

NHS Improvement (2008). *Delivering tomorrow's improvement agenda for the NHS.* www.improvement.nhs.uk (accessed 15 March 2010).

Nursing and Midwifery Council (2008). *The code: Standards of conduct, performance and ethics for nurses and midwives.* London: NMC.

Nutley, S. and Davies, H. (2000). Making a reality of evidence-based practice. In Davies, H.T.O., Nutley, S.M. and Smith, P.C. (eds.), *What works? Evidence-based policy and practice in public services* (pp. 317–50). Bristol: The Policy Press.

Onwujekwe, O., Onoka, C., Uzochukwu, B., Okoli, C., Obikeze, E. and Eze, S. (2009). Is community-based health insurance an equitable strategy for paying for healthcare? Experiences from southeast Nigeria. *Health Policy*, 92 (1), 96–102.

Parahoo, K. (2014). *Nursing research principles, process and issues* (3rd edn). Basingstoke: Palgrave Macmillan.

Perrotta, C., Ortiz, Z. and Rogue, M. (2005). *Chest physiotherapy for acute bronchiolitis in paediatric patients between 0 and 24 months old.* Oxford: The Cochrane Library.

Polit, D. and Beck, C. (2014). *Essentials of nursing research: Appraising evidence for nursing practice* (8th edn). Philadelphia, PA: Lippincott Williams and Wilkins.

Reason, P. and Bradbury, H. (eds) (2001). *Handbook of action research: Participative inquiry and practice* (Introduction, pp. 215–55). London: Sage.

Resuscitation Council (UK) (2010). *Resuscitation guidelines 2010.* www.resus.org.uk/pages/guide.htm (accessed 4 April 2014).

Robb, K., Wardle, J., Stubbings, S., Ramirez, A., Austoker, L., Macleod, U. et al. (2010). Ethnic disparities in knowledge of cancer screening programmes in the UK. *Journal of Medical Screening*, 17 (30), 125–31.

Robinson, L., Clare, L. and Evans, K. (2005). Making sense of dementia and adjusting to loss: psychological reactions to a diagnosis of dementia in couples. *Aging and Mental Health*, 9 (4), 337–47.

Rønnevig, M., Vandvik, P.O. and Bergbom, I. (2009). Patients' experiences of living with irritable bowel syndrome. *Journal of Advanced Nursing*, 65 (8), 1676–85.

Rycroft-Malone, J., Harvey, G., Kitson, A., McCormack, B., Seers, K. and Tichen, A. (2002) Getting evidence into practice: ingredients for change. *Nursing Standard*, 16 (37), 38–42.

Sackett, D.L., Straus, S.E., Richardson, W.S., Rosenberg, W. and Haynes, R.B. (2006). *Evidence-based medicine: How to practise and teach EBM* (2nd edn). Edinburgh: Churchill Livingstone.

Saflund, K. and Wredling, R. (2006). Differences within couples' experience of their hospital care and well-being three months after experiencing a stillbirth. *Acta Obstetrica et Gynecologica Scandinavica*, 85 (10), 1193–9.

Saurman, E., Perkins, D., Roberts, R., Robersts, A., Patfield, M. and Lyle, D. (2011) Responding to mental health emergencies; implementation of an innovative tele health service in rural and remote New South Wales. Australia. *Journal of Emergency Nursing*, 37 (5), 453–9.

Schmidt, N. and Brown, J. (2011). *Evidence based practice for nurses* (2nd edn). Sudbury, MA: Jones and Bartlett.

Schön, D. (1987). *Educating the reflective practitioner*. San Francisco, CA: Jossey Bass.

Scott, I. and Mazhindu, D. (2014). *Statistics for healthcare professionals: An introduction* (2nd edn). London: Sage.

Shaw, K., Brook, L., Cuddeford, L., Fitzmaurice, N., Thomas, C., Thompson, A. and Wallis, M. (2014). Prognostic indicators for children and young people at the end of life: a Delphi Study. *Palliative Medicine*, 28 (6), 501–12.

Silva, M., Viera, P., Countinho, S., Minderico, C., Matois, M., Sardinha, L. and Teixeria, P. (2010). Using self-determination theory to promote physical activity and weight control: a randomized controlled trial in women. *Journal of Behavioural Medicine*, 33, 110–22.

Strauss, A. and Corbin, J. (1997). *Grounded theory in practice*. Thousand Oaks, CA: Sage.

Strauss, A. and Corbin, J. (1998). *Basics of qualitative research: Procedures and techniques for generating grounded theory* (2nd edn). Thousand Oaks, CA: Sage.

Thomson, D. (2011). Ethnography: a suitable approach for providing an inside perspective on the everyday life's of health professionals. *International Journal of Therapy and Rehabilitation*, 18 (1), 10–17.

Trinder, L. and Reynolds, S. (eds.) (2000). *Evidence-based practice: A critical appraisal.* Oxford: Blackwell Science.

UK Clinical Research Collaboration (2006). *Developing the best research professionals.* London: UKCRC. www.ukcrc.org/activities/research-workforce.aspx (accessed 15 March 2010).

van Manen, M. (1990). *Researching lived experience: Human science for an action sensitive pedagogy.* London: Althouse Press.

Vuorenmaa, M., Halme, N., Astedt-Kuri, P., Kaunonen, M. and Perala, M. (2013). The validity and reliability of the Finnish Family Empowerment Scale (FES): a survey of parents with small children. *Child: Care, Health and Development,* 40 (4), 597–606.

Whitehead, D. (2005). Empirical or tacit knowledge as a basis for theory development? *Journal of Clinical Nursing,* 14 (2), 143–144.

Whiting, M. (2014). What it means to be the parent of a child with a disability or complex health need. *Nursing Children and Young People,* 26 (5), 26–9.

Yee Chin, W., Chan, K., Lan, C., Wong, S., Fong, D., Lo, Y., Lam, T.-P. and Chiu, B. (2014). Detection and management of depression in adult primary care patients in Hong Kong: a cross-sectional survey conducted by a primary care practice-based research network. *BMC Family Practice,* 15 (1), 30–52.

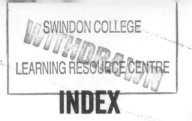

INDEX

Bold numbers refer to the glossary